Abe Hancock

Cookbook

ANTI-INFLAMMATORY DIET

for Arthritis

Easy and Delicious Recipes for Everyday Reduce Inflammation Processes in Joints Strengthen the Immune System and Improving Health

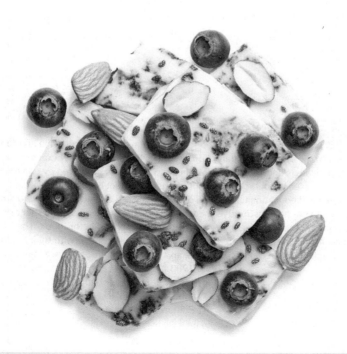

Disclaimer

The information presented in this cookbook is based on the author's research, knowledge, and experience. The recipes and guidelines provided are meant for general informational purposes only and are not intended to be a substitute for professional medical advice, diagnosis, or treatment. The author and publisher are not medical professionals, nutritionists, or dietitians, and the content of this book should not be used as a replacement for the advice of a qualified healthcare provider.

Before beginning any new diet, exercise program, or using any dietary supplements, it is strongly recommended that you consult with your healthcare provider, especially if you have any pre-existing health conditions, are pregnant, nursing, or taking medication. Every individual's health situation is unique, and it is important to base any dietary changes on your own health needs and goals.

The author and publisher disclaim any liability or responsibility for any adverse effects, reactions, or consequences resulting from the use or application of any recipes, advice, or suggestions contained in this book. The results of following the Anti-Inflammatory Diet will vary from person to person, and no specific outcomes, including weight loss or health improvements, are guaranteed.

All trademarks, service marks, and brand names mentioned in this book are the property of their respective owners, and no claim is made to such marks or names. References to any specific products, services, or processes do not constitute or imply an endorsement by the author or publisher.

ISBN: 9798342472272
Published by: Independently published
Printed in the United States of America
First Edition, 2024

TABLE OF CONTENS

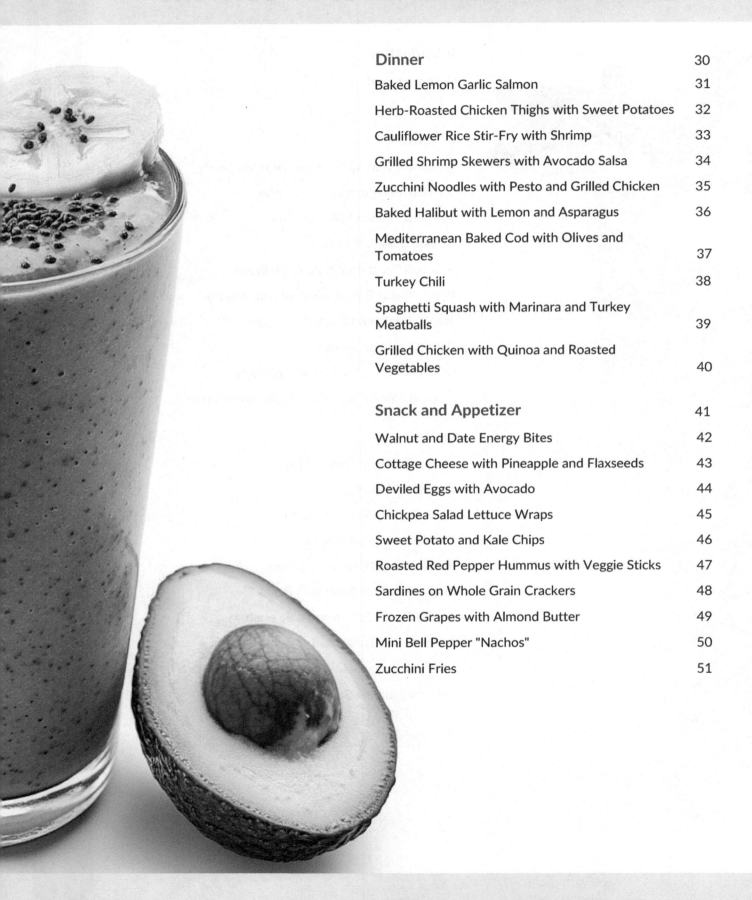

TABLE OF CONTENS

TABLE OF CONTENS

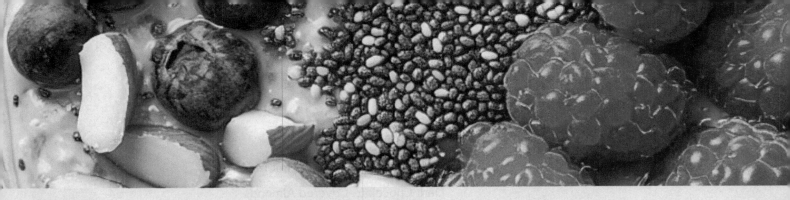

INTRODUCTION

Understanding Inflammation and Arthritis
Inflammation is a natural response of the body's immune system to protect against injury and infection. However, when inflammation becomes chronic, it can lead to various health issues, including arthritis. Arthritis is characterized by inflammation of the joints, causing pain, swelling, and stiffness. There are several types of arthritis, with osteoarthritis and rheumatoid arthritis being the most common. Understanding the connection between inflammation and arthritis is crucial for managing symptoms and improving overall quality of life.

Research has shown that certain foods can exacerbate inflammation, while others can help reduce it. By making informed dietary choices, individuals with arthritis can take an active role in managing their symptoms and promoting joint health.

Benefits of an Anti-Inflammatory Diet
An anti-inflammatory diet focuses on consuming foods that are known to reduce inflammation in the body. This approach not only aids in managing arthritis symptoms but also offers a multitude of health benefits, including:

- **Pain Reduction**: Many anti-inflammatory foods contain compounds that help alleviate pain and reduce swelling, making them beneficial for those with arthritis.
- **Improved Mobility**: A diet rich in anti-inflammatory ingredients can enhance joint function and mobility, allowing for better physical activity and overall well-being.
- **Enhanced Immune Function**: An anti-inflammatory diet supports the immune system, helping the body fend off illnesses and maintain optimal health.
- **Weight Management**: By focusing on nutrient-dense foods, this diet can assist in maintaining a healthy weight, which is particularly important for individuals with arthritis, as excess weight puts additional stress on joints.

- **Overall Health Improvement**: Beyond joint health, an anti-inflammatory diet promotes heart health, digestive health, and brain function, contributing to a higher quality of life.

How to Use This Cookbook
This cookbook is designed to be your comprehensive guide to embracing an anti-inflammatory lifestyle. Here's how to make the most of it:

- **Explore the Recipes**: With a wide range of delicious, easy-to-follow recipes, you'll find meals for every occasion. Feel free to experiment with different dishes and ingredients to discover what you enjoy most.
- **Track Your Progress**: Consider keeping a food journal to note how different meals affect your symptoms. This can help you identify which foods work best for you and enhance your overall experience with the anti-inflammatory diet.
- **Embrace the Journey**: Transitioning to an anti-inflammatory diet is not just about food; it's about cultivating a healthier relationship with what you eat. Be patient with yourself and enjoy the process of exploring new flavors and ingredients.

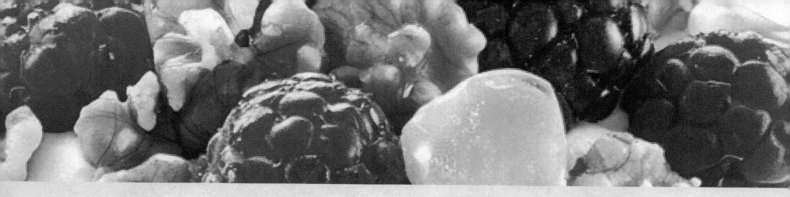

GETTING STARTED

Embarking on an anti-inflammatory diet can be a transformative journey toward better health, especially for those managing arthritis. This chapter is designed to help you establish a strong foundation for your new eating habits by outlining what to include in your pantry, foods to avoid, and essential kitchen tools that will make cooking enjoyable and efficient.

What to Include in Your Anti-Inflammatory Pantry

A well-stocked pantry is key to successfully following an anti-inflammatory diet. Focus on filling your shelves with nutrient-dense foods that fight inflammation. Here's a list of essentials:

- **Whole Grains**: Quinoa, brown rice, oats, and whole wheat products provide fiber and essential nutrients.
- **Fruits and Vegetables**: Fresh, frozen, or canned (without added sugar or salt) options are great. Focus on berries, leafy greens, cruciferous vegetables (like broccoli and kale), and colorful produce.
- **Healthy Fats**: Extra virgin olive oil, avocados, nuts (almonds, walnuts), and seeds (chia, flaxseed) are excellent sources of omega-3 fatty acids and antioxidants.
- **Legumes**: Beans, lentils, and chickpeas are not only protein-rich but also packed with fiber and phytonutrients.
- **Herbs and Spices**: Stock your pantry with anti-inflammatory herbs and spices like turmeric, ginger, garlic, cinnamon, and basil. These not only add flavor but also provide significant health benefits.
- **Lean Proteins**: Incorporate skinless poultry, fatty fish (like salmon), and plant-based proteins to support muscle health without contributing to inflammation.

Foods to Avoid

Just as important as knowing what to include in your diet is being aware of what to avoid. Certain foods can trigger inflammation and exacerbate symptoms of arthritis. Here are the main culprits to limit or eliminate:

- **Processed Foods**: Fast food, sugary snacks, and ready-to-eat meals often contain unhealthy fats, sugars, and preservatives that can increase inflammation.
- **Refined Carbohydrates**: White bread, pastries, and other processed grains can spike blood sugar levels and contribute to inflammatory responses.
- **Sugary Beverages**: Soda, sweetened teas, and energy drinks are high in sugar and can lead to increased inflammation.
- **Excessive Alcohol**: While moderate consumption may be acceptable, excessive alcohol intake can lead to inflammation and health issues.
- **Trans Fats**: Found in many fried and baked goods, these unhealthy fats are known to promote inflammation.
- **Certain Vegetable Oils**: Oils high in omega-6 fatty acids (such as corn and soybean oil) should be limited, as they can contribute to inflammation.

Essential Kitchen Tools

Having the right kitchen tools can make meal preparation more efficient and enjoyable. Here are some essential items to consider:

- **Good Quality Chef's Knife**: A sharp knife is crucial for cutting fruits, vegetables, and proteins with ease.
- **Cutting Boards**: Invest in a couple of sturdy cutting boards—preferably one for vegetables and another for proteins to avoid cross-contamination.
- **Food Processor or Blender**: Great for making smoothies, soups, and sauces quickly and easily.
- **Measuring Cups and Spoons**: Essential for accurately measuring ingredients, especially when following recipes.
- **Non-Stick Cookware**: Look for high-quality non-stick pans that allow for healthier cooking with less oil.
- **Slow Cooker or Instant Pot**: These appliances are perfect for preparing flavorful, nutrient-rich meals with minimal effort.
- **Storage Containers**: Use glass or BPA-free plastic containers to store leftovers and meal prep items efficiently.

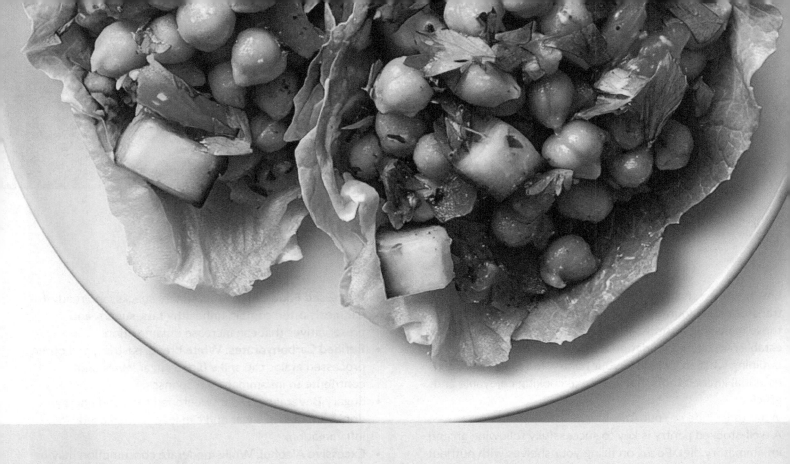

BREAKFAST

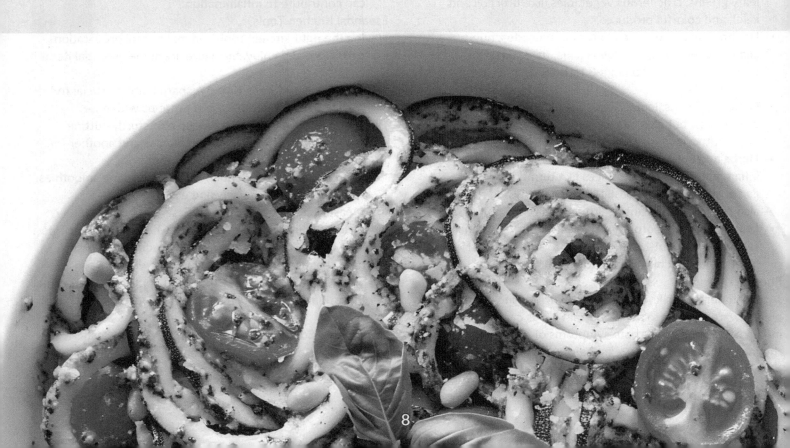

OVERNIGHT OATS WITH BERRIES AND CHIA SEEDS

COOK TIME: 10 MIN   SERVICE: 2 PERSONS

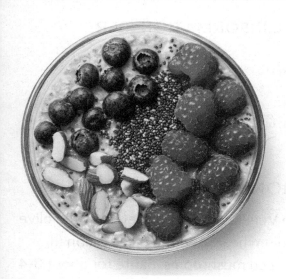

INGREDIENTS

- **1 cup rolled oats**
- **2 cups unsweetened almond milk (or any plant-based milk)**
- **2 tablespoons chia seeds**
- **1 tablespoon maple syrup (optional, adjust to taste)**
- **1 teaspoon vanilla extract**
- **1 cup mixed fresh berries (strawberries, blueberries, raspberries)**
- **1/4 cup sliced almonds or walnuts (optional, for topping)**

NUTRITIONAL INFORMATION (PER SERVING)

- Calories: 300 kcal
- Protein: 8g
- Fat: 10g
- Carbohydrates: 45g
- Fiber: 10g

INSTRUCTIONS

1. Combine Ingredients: In a mixing bowl, combine the rolled oats, almond milk, chia seeds, maple syrup, and vanilla extract. Stir well to ensure all ingredients are mixed thoroughly.
2. Refrigerate: Divide the mixture evenly between two jars or bowls. Cover and refrigerate overnight (or for at least 4 hours) to allow the oats and chia seeds to absorb the liquid and thicken.
3. Add Toppings: In the morning, give the oats a good stir. Top with mixed fresh berries and nuts (if using) before serving.
4. Serve: Enjoy cold or heat briefly in the microwave if you prefer warm oats.

SPINACH AND MUSHROOM OMELETTE

COOK TIME: **20 MIN**   SERVICE: **2 PERSONS**

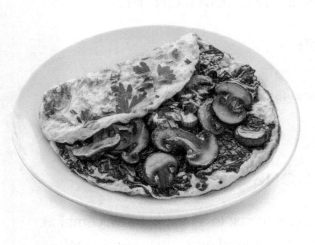

NUTRITIONAL INFORMATION (PER SERVING)

- Calories: 230 kcal
- Protein: 14g
- Fat: 16g
- Carbohydrates: 6g
- Fiber: 1g

INGREDIENTS

- **4 large eggs**
- **1 cup fresh spinach, chopped**
- **1/2 cup mushrooms, sliced (cremini or button)**
- **1/4 cup onion, diced (optional)**
- **1 tablespoon olive oil**
- **Salt and pepper to taste**
- **1/4 teaspoon turmeric (optional, for added anti-inflammatory benefits)**
- **Fresh herbs for garnish (parsley or chives, optional)**

INSTRUCTIONS

1. Prepare the Vegetables: In a skillet, heat the olive oil over medium heat. Add the diced onion (if using) and sliced mushrooms. Sauté for about 3-4 minutes, or until the mushrooms are soft and the onions are translucent.
2. Add Spinach: Add the chopped spinach to the skillet and sauté for an additional 1-2 minutes, until the spinach is wilted. If using turmeric, add it during this step. Season with salt and pepper to taste. Remove the vegetable mixture from the skillet and set aside.
3. Whisk the Eggs: In a bowl, whisk the eggs until well combined. Season with a pinch of salt and pepper.
4. Cook the Omelette: In the same skillet, add a little more olive oil if necessary and pour in the whisked eggs, swirling the pan to evenly coat the bottom. Cook for about 2-3 minutes, or until the edges start to set.
5. Add the Filling: Once the eggs are mostly set, spoon the spinach and mushroom mixture onto one half of the omelette. Allow it to cook for another minute, then gently fold the omelette over the filling.
6. Serve: Cook for an additional minute, then slide the omelette onto a plate. Garnish with fresh herbs if desired. Serve immediately.

TURMERIC GOLDEN MILK SMOOTHIE

COOK TIME: **5 MIN**   SERVICE: **2 PERSONS**

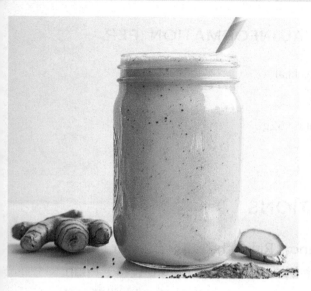

INGREDIENTS

- **1 cup unsweetened almond milk (or any plant-based milk)**
- **1 medium banana (frozen for a creamier texture)**
- **1 tablespoon turmeric powder**
- **1 teaspoon fresh ginger, grated (or 1/2 teaspoon ginger powder)**
- **1 tablespoon honey or maple syrup (adjust to taste)**
- **1/4 teaspoon black pepper (enhances turmeric absorption)**
- **1 tablespoon chia seeds (optional, for added fiber)**
- **1/2 teaspoon cinnamon (optional, for flavor)**
- **Ice cubes (optional, for a colder smoothie)**

NUTRITIONAL INFORMATION (PER SERVING)

- Calories: 180 kcal
- Protein: 4g
- Fat: 5g
- Carbohydrates: 32g
- Fiber: 5g

INSTRUCTIONS

1. Blend Ingredients: In a blender, combine the almond milk, banana, turmeric powder, ginger, honey or maple syrup, black pepper, chia seeds, and cinnamon (if using).
2. Adjust Consistency: If you prefer a colder smoothie, add a handful of ice cubes.
3. Blend Until Smooth: Blend on high until all ingredients are well combined and the smoothie is creamy.
4. Serve: Pour the smoothie into two glasses and enjoy immediately.

QUINOA BREAKFAST BOWL

COOK TIME: **25 MIN**   SERVICE: **2 PERSONS**

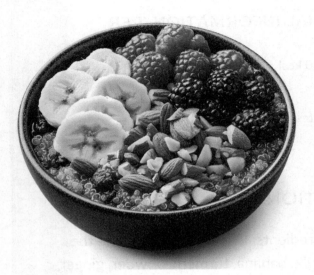

INGREDIENTS

- **1 cup quinoa (uncooked)**
- **2 cups water or unsweetened almond milk**
- **1 medium banana, sliced**
- **1/2 cup mixed berries (fresh or frozen)**
- **1/4 cup chopped nuts (walnuts or almonds)**
- **1 tablespoon chia seeds**
- **1 tablespoon honey or maple syrup (optional, adjust to taste)**
- **1/2 teaspoon cinnamon**
- **Pinch of salt**

NUTRITIONAL INFORMATION (PER SERVING)

- Calories: 350 kcal
- Protein: 10g
- Fat: 14g
- Carbohydrates: 52g
- Fiber: 10g

INSTRUCTIONS

1. Cook Quinoa: Rinse the quinoa under cold water to remove bitterness. In a medium saucepan, combine quinoa, water (or almond milk), and a pinch of salt. Bring to a boil over medium-high heat. Once boiling, reduce the heat to low, cover, and simmer for about 15 minutes, or until the quinoa is fluffy and the liquid is absorbed.
2. Prepare Toppings: While the quinoa cooks, prepare your toppings. Slice the banana, and if using frozen berries, allow them to thaw slightly.
3. Assemble Bowls: Once the quinoa is cooked, divide it evenly between two bowls. Top each bowl with sliced banana, mixed berries, chopped nuts, chia seeds, honey or maple syrup (if using), and a sprinkle of cinnamon.
4. Serve: Enjoy your nutritious quinoa breakfast bowl warm or at room temperature.

AVOCADO TOAST ON WHOLE GRAIN BREAD

COOK TIME: **10 MIN**   SERVICE: **2 PERSONS**

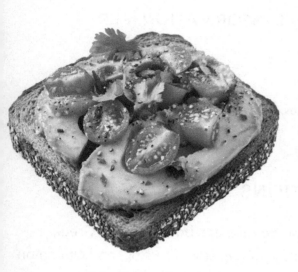

INGREDIENTS

- **2 slices whole grain bread (or gluten-free bread)**
- **1 ripe avocado**
- **1 tablespoon lemon juice**
- **Salt and pepper to taste**
- **1/4 teaspoon red pepper flakes (optional, for a bit of heat)**
- **1/4 cup cherry tomatoes, halved (optional, for topping)**
- **Fresh herbs (such as cilantro or parsley, for garnish)**

NUTRITIONAL INFORMATION (PER SERVING)

- Calories: 250 kcal
- Protein: 6g
- Fat: 14g
- Carbohydrates: 28g
- Fiber: 10g

INSTRUCTIONS

1. Toast the Bread: Toast the whole grain bread slices in a toaster or on a skillet until golden brown and crispy.
2. Prepare the Avocado: While the bread is toasting, cut the avocado in half, remove the pit, and scoop the flesh into a bowl. Add lemon juice, salt, and pepper, and mash the avocado with a fork until creamy but still slightly chunky.
3. Assemble the Toast: Once the bread is toasted, spread the mashed avocado evenly over each slice.
4. Add Toppings: If using, sprinkle red pepper flakes over the avocado toast and top with halved cherry tomatoes. Garnish with fresh herbs for added flavor.
5. Serve: Enjoy your delicious avocado toast immediately while the bread is still warm.

GREEK YOGURT PARFAIT WITH NUTS AND HONEY

COOK TIME: **5 MIN**   SERVICE: **2 PERSONS**

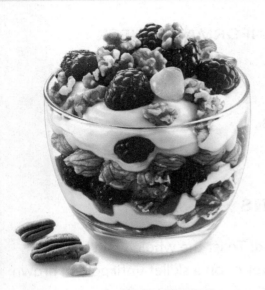

INGREDIENTS

- **2 cups plain Greek yogurt (preferably low-fat or non-fat)**
- **1/2 cup mixed berries (fresh or frozen)**
- **1/4 cup nuts (walnuts, almonds, or pecans), chopped**
- **2 tablespoons honey (or maple syrup, if preferred)**
- **1/2 teaspoon vanilla extract (optional)**
- **1/4 teaspoon cinnamon (optional, for added flavor)**

NUTRITIONAL INFORMATION (PER SERVING)

- Calories: 300 kcal
- Protein: 20g
- Fat: 12g
- Carbohydrates: 34g
- Fiber: 5g

INSTRUCTIONS

1. Prepare the Yogurt: In a bowl, mix the Greek yogurt with vanilla extract (if using) and cinnamon (if desired). This adds extra flavor to your yogurt.
2. Layer the Ingredients: In two serving glasses or bowls, layer half of the yogurt at the bottom. Add a layer of mixed berries, followed by a layer of chopped nuts.
3. Repeat the Layers: Add the remaining yogurt on top, followed by another layer of berries and nuts.
4. Drizzle with Honey: Finish by drizzling honey (or maple syrup) on top of each parfait.
5. Serve: Enjoy immediately as a nutritious breakfast or snack.

SWEET POTATO AND BLACK BEAN HASH

COOK TIME: **30 MIN**   SERVICE: **2 PERSONS**

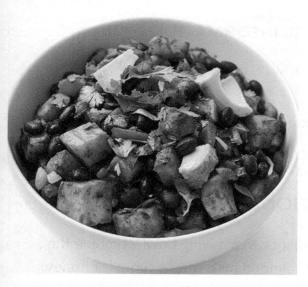

INGREDIENTS

- 1 medium sweet potato, peeled and diced (about 1 cup)
- 1 can (15 oz) black beans, drained and rinsed
- 1/2 bell pepper (red or yellow), diced
- 1/4 onion, diced
- 2 tablespoons olive oil
- 1 teaspoon cumin
- 1/2 teaspoon smoked paprika
- Salt and pepper to taste
- Fresh cilantro or parsley for garnish (optional)
- 1 avocado, sliced (optional, for serving)

NUTRITIONAL INFORMATION (PER SERVING)

- Calories: 350 kcal
- Protein: 12g
- Fat: 14g
- Carbohydrates: 52g
- Fiber: 12g

INSTRUCTIONS

1. Cook Sweet Potatoes: In a large skillet, heat 1 tablespoon of olive oil over medium heat. Add the diced sweet potatoes and cook for about 10 minutes, stirring occasionally, until they are tender and slightly crispy.
2. Add Vegetables: Add the diced onion and bell pepper to the skillet. Sauté for an additional 5 minutes, or until the vegetables are softened.
3. Season and Add Black Beans: Stir in the black beans, cumin, smoked paprika, salt, and pepper. Cook for another 2-3 minutes, allowing the beans to warm through and the flavors to meld.
4. Serve: Divide the hash between two plates. Garnish with fresh cilantro or parsley if desired, and serve with sliced avocado for added creaminess.

BERRY CHIA SEED PUDDING

COOK TIME: 10 MIN **CHILLING TIME: 2 HOURS (OR OVERNIGHT)**
SERVICE: 2 PERSONS

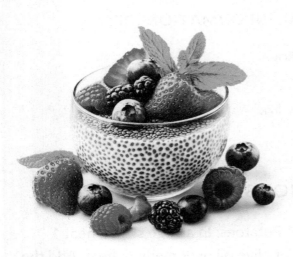

NUTRITIONAL INFORMATION (PER SERVING)

- Calories: 250 kcal
- Protein: 8g
- Fat: 12g
- Carbohydrates: 32g
- Fiber: 10g

INGREDIENTS

- 1/2 cup chia seeds
- 2 cups unsweetened almond milk (or any plant-based milk)
- 1 tablespoon maple syrup or honey (adjust to taste)
- 1 teaspoon vanilla extract
- 1 cup mixed berries (fresh or frozen; strawberries, blueberries, raspberries)
- Fresh mint leaves for garnish (optional)

INSTRUCTIONS

1. Mix Ingredients: In a mixing bowl, combine the chia seeds, almond milk, maple syrup (or honey), and vanilla extract. Stir well to ensure the chia seeds are evenly distributed.
2. Refrigerate: Pour the mixture into two serving jars or bowls. Cover and refrigerate for at least 2 hours, or overnight, to allow the chia seeds to absorb the liquid and thicken into a pudding-like consistency.
3. Serve: Once chilled, give the pudding a good stir. Top each serving with mixed berries and garnish with fresh mint leaves if desired.
4. Enjoy: Serve chilled as a healthy breakfast or snack.

OATMEAL WITH CINNAMON AND WALNUTS

COOK TIME: **15** MIN   SERVICE: **2 PERSONS**

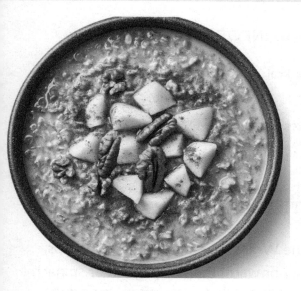

INGREDIENTS

- **1 cup rolled oats**
- **2 cups water or unsweetened almond milk**
- **1/2 teaspoon cinnamon (plus extra for topping)**
- **1/4 teaspoon salt**
- **1/2 cup walnuts, chopped**
- **1 tablespoon maple syrup or honey (optional, adjust to taste)**
- **1 medium apple, diced (optional, for added sweetness and nutrition)**

NUTRITIONAL INFORMATION (PER SERVING)

- Calories: 320 kcal
- Protein: 10g
- Fat: 14g
- Carbohydrates: 42g
- Fiber: 7g

INSTRUCTIONS

1. Cook Oats: In a medium saucepan, combine the rolled oats, water (or almond milk), cinnamon, and salt. Bring to a boil over medium-high heat.
2. Simmer: Once boiling, reduce the heat to low and simmer for about 5-7 minutes, stirring occasionally, until the oats are soft and have absorbed most of the liquid. If you prefer a creamier consistency, cook a bit longer or add more liquid.
3. Add Walnuts and Sweetener: Stir in the chopped walnuts and maple syrup (or honey), and mix well. If using, add the diced apple for additional sweetness.
4. Serve: Divide the oatmeal into two bowls. Top with extra walnuts and a sprinkle of cinnamon before serving.

SMOKED SALMON AND AVOCADO BREAKFAST WRAP

COOK TIME: **10** MIN   SERVICE: **2 PERSONS**

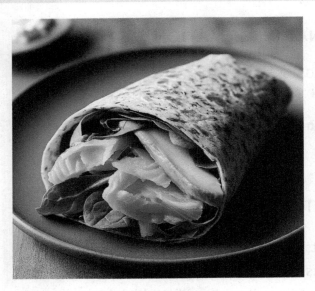

INGREDIENTS

- **2 whole grain or spinach wraps (or gluten-free wraps)**
- **4 ounces smoked salmon**
- **1 ripe avocado, sliced**
- **1/2 cup fresh spinach or arugula**
- **1/4 cup cream cheese or Greek yogurt (optional)**
- **1 tablespoon capers (optional)**
- **Fresh lemon juice (to taste)**
- **Salt and pepper to taste**

NUTRITIONAL INFORMATION (PER SERVING)

- Calories: 350 kcal
- Protein: 20g
- Fat: 20g
- Carbohydrates: 30g
- Fiber: 8g

INSTRUCTIONS

1. Prepare the Wraps: If you prefer warm wraps, lightly toast or warm the whole grain or spinach wraps in a skillet over low heat for about 1-2 minutes on each side.
2. Assemble the Wrap: Lay each wrap flat on a clean surface. Spread a layer of cream cheese or Greek yogurt over each wrap, if using.
3. Layer Ingredients: On each wrap, arrange the sliced avocado, smoked salmon, and fresh spinach or arugula. If desired, add capers for extra flavor.
4. Season: Drizzle a little fresh lemon juice over the filling and season with salt and pepper to taste.
5. Wrap It Up: Fold in the sides of the wrap and then roll it up tightly from the bottom to the top. Slice in half diagonally.
6. Serve: Enjoy your smoked salmon and avocado breakfast wrap immediately!

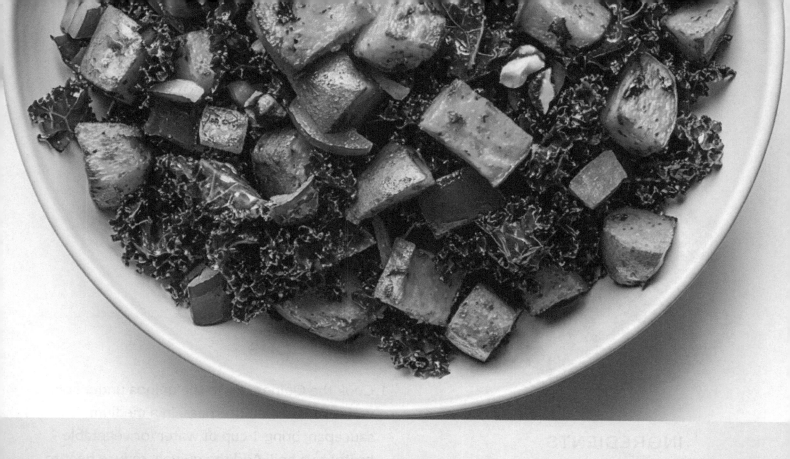

Lunch

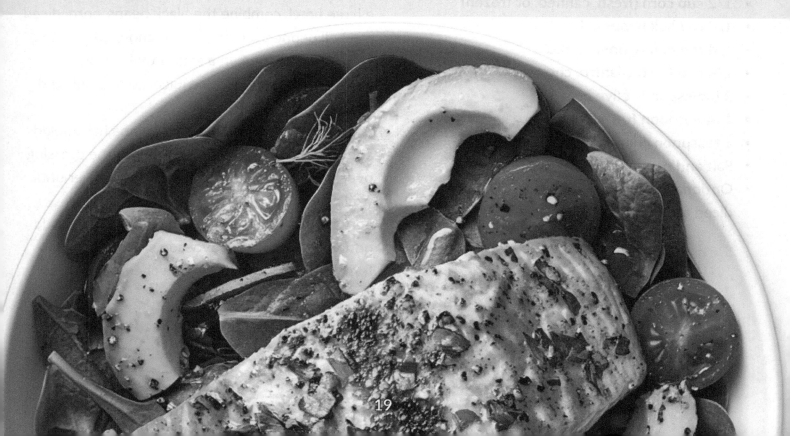

QUINOA AND BLACK BEAN SALAD

COOK TIME: **25 MIN**   SERVICE: **2 PERSONS**

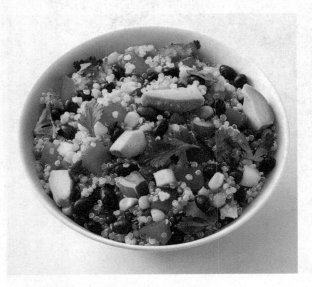

NUTRITIONAL INFORMATION (PER SERVING)

- Calories: 350 kcal
- Protein: 12g
- Fat: 14g
- Carbohydrates: 47g
- Fiber: 12g

INGREDIENTS

- 1/2 cup quinoa (uncooked)
- 1 cup water or vegetable broth (for extra flavor)
- 1 can (15 oz) black beans, drained and rinsed
- 1/2 cup corn (fresh, canned, or frozen)
- 1/2 red bell pepper, diced
- 1/4 red onion, finely diced
- 1/4 cup fresh cilantro, chopped
- 2 tablespoons olive oil
- 1 tablespoon fresh lime juice
- 1 teaspoon cumin
- Salt and pepper to taste
- Optional toppings: avocado slices, diced tomatoes, or feta cheese

INSTRUCTIONS

1. Cook the Quinoa: Rinse the quinoa under cold water to remove bitterness. In a medium saucepan, bring 1 cup of water (or vegetable broth) to a boil. Add the quinoa, reduce heat to low, cover, and simmer for about 12-15 minutes, or until the quinoa has absorbed all the liquid and is tender. Fluff with a fork and set aside to cool slightly.
2. Prepare the Salad: While the quinoa is cooking, in a large bowl, combine the black beans, corn, diced red bell pepper, red onion, and chopped cilantro.
3. Make the Dressing: In a small bowl, whisk together the olive oil, lime juice, cumin, salt, and pepper.
4. Assemble the Salad: Once the quinoa has cooled, add it to the vegetable mixture. Pour the dressing over the salad and toss everything together until well combined.
5. Serve: Divide the salad between two plates. Add optional toppings like avocado slices, diced tomatoes, or a sprinkle of feta cheese if desired.

TURMERIC CHICKEN SALAD

COOK TIME: **30 MIN**   SERVICE: **2 PERSONS**

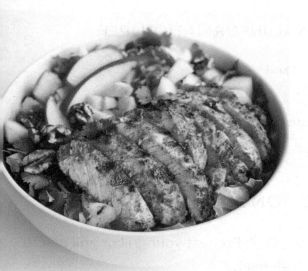

NUTRITIONAL INFORMATION (PER SERVING)

- Calories: 420 kcal
- Protein: 40g
- Fat: 22g
- Carbohydrates: 20g
- Fiber: 4g

INGREDIENTS

- **2 boneless, skinless chicken breasts (about 8 oz each)**
- **1 teaspoon turmeric powder**
- **1/2 teaspoon ground cumin**
- **1/2 teaspoon garlic powder**
- **Salt and pepper to taste**
- **1 tablespoon olive oil**
- **1/4 cup plain Greek yogurt (or dairy-free yogurt)**
- **1 tablespoon lemon juice**
- **1 apple, diced**
- **1/4 cup walnuts, chopped**
- **1/4 cup celery, chopped**
- **Fresh cilantro or parsley for garnish (optional)**

INSTRUCTIONS

1. Season the Chicken: Rub the chicken breasts with turmeric, cumin, garlic powder, salt, and pepper. Set aside while you heat the skillet.
2. Cook the Chicken: In a large skillet, heat the olive oil over medium heat. Add the seasoned chicken breasts and cook for about 6-8 minutes on each side, or until the internal temperature reaches 165°F (75°C). Once cooked, remove from the skillet and let it rest for 5 minutes. After resting, dice the chicken into bite-sized pieces.
3. Prepare the Salad: In a large bowl, combine the Greek yogurt and lemon juice. Stir in the diced apple, walnuts, and celery.
4. Assemble the Salad: Add the diced chicken to the bowl and mix until all ingredients are well coated. Adjust the seasoning with salt and pepper, if needed.
5. Serve: Divide the salad between two plates. Garnish with fresh cilantro or parsley if desired. Enjoy immediately or refrigerate for up to 2 days.

ZESTY GRILLED VEGETABLE SALAD

COOK TIME: 25 MIN   SERVICE: 2 PERSONS

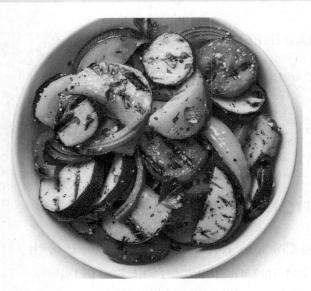

INGREDIENTS

- 1 zucchini, sliced lengthwise
- 1 red bell pepper, cut into quarters
- 1 yellow squash, sliced lengthwise
- 1 red onion, cut into thick slices
- 1 tablespoon olive oil
- Salt and pepper to taste
- 1/4 cup fresh cilantro or parsley, chopped (optional)
- 1/4 cup crumbled feta cheese (optional)
- 1 avocado, sliced (optional)

For the Dressing:
- 2 tablespoons olive oil
- 1 tablespoon fresh lemon juice
- 1 teaspoon Dijon mustard
- 1/2 teaspoon garlic powder
- 1/4 teaspoon ground cumin
- Salt and pepper to taste

NUTRITIONAL INFORMATION (PER SERVING)

- Calories: 270 kcal
- Protein: 5g
- Fat: 22g
- Carbohydrates: 18g
- Fiber: 7g

INSTRUCTIONS

1. Preheat the Grill: Preheat your grill or grill pan to medium-high heat.
2. Prepare the Vegetables: Brush the zucchini, bell pepper, yellow squash, and red onion slices with 1 tablespoon of olive oil. Season with salt and pepper.
3. Grill the Vegetables: Place the vegetables on the grill and cook for about 4-5 minutes per side, until they are tender and have nice grill marks. Once cooked, remove from the grill and let them cool slightly before cutting into bite-sized pieces.
4. Prepare the Dressing: In a small bowl, whisk together the olive oil, lemon juice, Dijon mustard, garlic powder, cumin, salt, and pepper until well combined.
5. Assemble the Salad: In a large salad bowl, toss the grilled vegetables with the dressing. Add in the fresh cilantro or parsley, crumbled feta cheese (if using), and sliced avocado (optional).
6. Serve: Divide the salad between two plates and enjoy immediately.

LENTIL AND VEGETABLE SOUP

COOK TIME: **40 MIN**   SERVICE: **2 PERSONS**

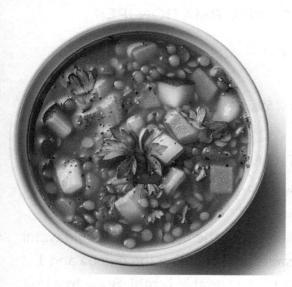

INGREDIENTS

- 1/2 cup dried green or brown lentils, rinsed
- 1 tablespoon olive oil
- 1/2 onion, diced
- 1 carrot, diced
- 1 celery stalk, diced
- 2 cloves garlic, minced
- 1/2 zucchini, diced
- 4 cups vegetable broth (low-sodium)
- 1/2 teaspoon ground turmeric
- 1/2 teaspoon cumin
- 1/2 teaspoon smoked paprika (optional)
- Salt and pepper to taste
- 1/4 cup fresh parsley, chopped (optional, for garnish)
- 1 tablespoon lemon juice (optional, for serving)

NUTRITIONAL INFORMATION (PER SERVING)

- Calories: 300 kcal
- Protein: 12g
- Fat: 6g
- Carbohydrates: 45g
- Fiber: 14g

INSTRUCTIONS

1. Sauté the Vegetables: In a large pot, heat the olive oil over medium heat. Add the diced onion, carrot, and celery, and sauté for 5 minutes until softened. Add the minced garlic and sauté for an additional 1 minute until fragrant.
2. Add Lentils and Spices: Stir in the lentils, turmeric, cumin, and smoked paprika (if using). Cook for another 1-2 minutes to coat the lentils and spices.
3. Add Broth and Vegetables: Pour in the vegetable broth and add the diced zucchini. Bring the soup to a boil, then reduce the heat to low and simmer for 25-30 minutes, or until the lentils are tender.
4. Season and Serve: Once the lentils are cooked, season the soup with salt and pepper to taste. Stir in the fresh parsley and a splash of lemon juice for added brightness.
5. Serve: Divide the soup into two bowls and enjoy hot.

ROASTED VEGETABLE QUINOA BOWL

COOK TIME: 35 MIN   SERVICE: 2 PERSONS

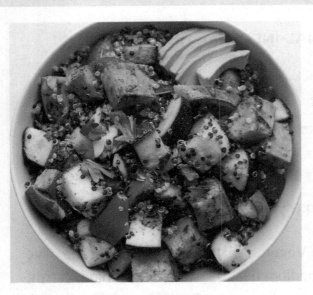

NUTRITIONAL INFORMATION (PER SERVING)

- Calories: 380 kcal
- Protein: 10g
- Fat: 18g
- Carbohydrates: 50g
- Fiber: 9g

INGREDIENTS

- 1/2 cup quinoa, uncooked
- 1 cup water or vegetable broth (for cooking quinoa)
- 1 zucchini, diced
- 1 red bell pepper, diced
- 1 sweet potato, peeled and diced
- 1/2 red onion, sliced
- 2 tablespoons olive oil
- 1 teaspoon smoked paprika
- 1 teaspoon ground cumin
- Salt and pepper to taste
- 1 tablespoon fresh lemon juice
- 1/4 cup fresh parsley or cilantro, chopped (optional for garnish)
- 1/4 cup tahini (optional, for drizzle)
- 1/2 avocado, sliced (optional, for topping)

INSTRUCTIONS

1. Preheat Oven: Preheat your oven to 400°F (200°C).
2. Cook Quinoa: Rinse the quinoa under cold water. In a small saucepan, combine the quinoa and 1 cup of water (or vegetable broth). Bring to a boil, reduce the heat to low, cover, and simmer for 12-15 minutes, or until the quinoa has absorbed the liquid. Fluff with a fork and set aside.
3. Prepare Vegetables: While the quinoa is cooking, toss the diced zucchini, red bell pepper, sweet potato, and red onion with olive oil, smoked paprika, cumin, salt, and pepper on a baking sheet.
4. Roast Vegetables: Spread the vegetables in a single layer on the baking sheet. Roast for 20-25 minutes, or until the vegetables are tender and slightly caramelized, stirring halfway through for even cooking.
5. Assemble the Bowl: Once the vegetables are roasted and the quinoa is cooked, divide the quinoa into two bowls. Top each bowl with the roasted vegetables.
6. Add Toppings: Drizzle with lemon juice and garnish with fresh parsley or cilantro. For additional flavor, drizzle tahini over the top and add sliced avocado if desired.
7. Serve: Enjoy your warm, nutritious quinoa bowl immediately.

ZUCCHINI NOODLE SALAD WITH PESTO

COOK TIME: **10 MIN**   SERVICE: **2 PERSONS**

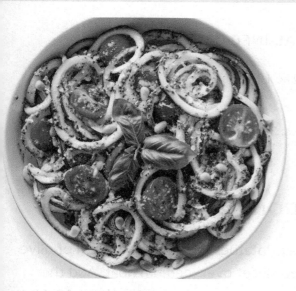

INGREDIENTS

- **2 medium zucchini, spiralized into noodles (or use a vegetable peeler to make thin strips)**
- **1/4 cup pesto (store-bought or homemade, preferably made with olive oil)**
- **1/2 cup cherry tomatoes, halved**
- **1/4 cup pine nuts (optional, for added crunch)**
- **2 tablespoons grated Parmesan cheese (optional, for serving)**
- **1 tablespoon lemon juice**
- **Salt and pepper to taste**
- **Fresh basil leaves for garnish (optional)**

NUTRITIONAL INFORMATION (PER SERVING)

- Calories: 220 kcal
- Protein: 5g
- Fat: 18g
- Carbohydrates: 11g
- Fiber: 4g

INSTRUCTIONS

1. Prepare the Zucchini Noodles: Spiralize the zucchini using a spiralizer or use a vegetable peeler to create thin strips. Place the zucchini noodles in a large mixing bowl.
2. Add Ingredients: Add the cherry tomatoes, pesto, lemon juice, and pine nuts to the zucchini noodles. Season with salt and pepper to taste.
3. Toss to Combine: Gently toss the salad until all the ingredients are evenly coated with the pesto.
4. Serve: Divide the salad between two plates. Garnish with grated Parmesan cheese and fresh basil leaves if desired. Serve immediately.

SAVORY SWEET POTATO AND KALE HASH

COOK TIME: 30 MIN   SERVICE: 2 PERSONS

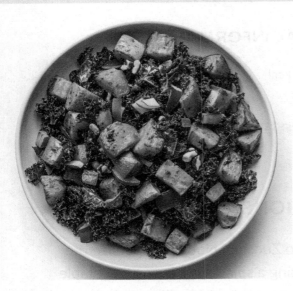

INGREDIENTS

- 1 large sweet potato, peeled and diced
- 1 tablespoon olive oil
- 1/2 red onion, diced
- 1 clove garlic, minced
- 2 cups fresh kale, chopped (stems removed)
- 1/2 teaspoon smoked paprika
- 1/4 teaspoon ground cumin
- Salt and pepper to taste
- 1/4 cup chopped walnuts (optional, for added crunch)
- 1 tablespoon fresh lemon juice (optional, for garnish)

NUTRITIONAL INFORMATION (PER SERVING)

- Calories: 280 kcal
- Protein: 5g
- Fat: 14g
- Carbohydrates: 38g
- Fiber: 7g

INSTRUCTIONS

1. Cook Sweet Potatoes: Heat 1 tablespoon of olive oil in a large skillet over medium heat. Add the diced sweet potatoes and cook for about 10-12 minutes, stirring occasionally, until they are tender and slightly crispy.
2. Add Onion and Garlic: Add the diced red onion and minced garlic to the skillet. Cook for 3-4 minutes until the onions are soft and fragrant.
3. Add Kale: Stir in the chopped kale and cook for another 3-4 minutes until the kale is wilted and tender.
4. Season: Sprinkle the smoked paprika, ground cumin, salt, and pepper over the hash. Stir well to combine and cook for another 1-2 minutes to let the flavors meld.
5. Optional Toppings: If using, sprinkle chopped walnuts on top for added crunch and drizzle with fresh lemon juice for a bright, zesty flavor.
6. Serve: Divide the sweet potato and kale hash between two plates and enjoy immediately.

AVOCADO AND TUNA SALAD

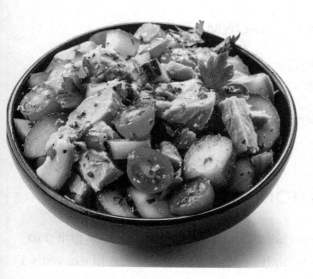

NUTRITIONAL INFORMATION (PER SERVING)

- Calories: 350 kcal
- Protein: 24g
- Fat: 24g
- Carbohydrates: 12g
- Fiber: 6g

INGREDIENTS

- **1 can (5 oz) tuna in water, drained**
- **1 ripe avocado, diced**
- **1 tablespoon olive oil**
- **1 tablespoon lemon juice**
- **1/4 cup red onion, finely chopped**
- **1/2 cup cucumber, diced**
- **1/2 cup cherry tomatoes, halved**
- **Salt and pepper to taste**
- **Fresh parsley or cilantro for garnish (optional)**

INSTRUCTIONS

1. Prepare the Ingredients: In a medium bowl, combine the drained tuna, diced avocado, red onion, cucumber, and cherry tomatoes.
2. Make the Dressing: In a small bowl, whisk together the olive oil, lemon juice, salt, and pepper.
3. Toss the Salad: Pour the dressing over the tuna and avocado mixture. Gently toss everything together until well combined. Be careful not to mash the avocado too much.
4. Serve: Divide the salad between two plates and garnish with fresh parsley or cilantro, if desired.

GRILLED SALMON SALAD WITH AVOCADO AND SPINACH

COOK TIME: **20 MIN**   SERVICE: **2 PERSONS**

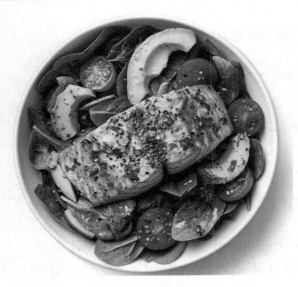

INGREDIENTS

- **2 salmon fillets (about 4 oz each)**
- **1 tablespoon olive oil**
- **Salt and pepper to taste**
- **1/2 teaspoon garlic powder**
- **1/2 teaspoon paprika**
- **4 cups fresh spinach leaves**
- **1 avocado, sliced**
- **1/2 cup cherry tomatoes, halved**
- **1/4 red onion, thinly sliced**
- **1 tablespoon lemon juice**
- **2 tablespoons olive oil (for dressing)**
- **Salt and pepper (for dressing)**
- **Fresh dill or parsley for garnish (optional)**

NUTRITIONAL INFORMATION (PER SERVING)

- Calories: 460 kcal
- Protein: 30g
- Fat: 35g
- Carbohydrates: 12g
- Fiber: 7g

INSTRUCTIONS

1. Prepare the Salmon: Preheat your grill or grill pan to medium-high heat. Rub the salmon fillets with 1 tablespoon of olive oil, and season with salt, pepper, garlic powder, and paprika.
2. Grill the Salmon: Place the salmon fillets on the grill, skin-side down, and cook for about 4-5 minutes on each side, or until the salmon is cooked through and flakes easily with a fork. Remove from the grill and set aside.
3. Prepare the Salad: While the salmon is grilling, divide the spinach leaves between two plates. Top with sliced avocado, cherry tomatoes, and red onion.
4. Make the Dressing: In a small bowl, whisk together the lemon juice, 2 tablespoons of olive oil, salt, and pepper.
5. Assemble the Salad: Once the salmon has slightly cooled, place one fillet on top of each salad. Drizzle with the lemon-olive oil dressing and garnish with fresh dill or parsley if desired.
6. Serve: Enjoy this light, refreshing salad immediately while the salmon is still warm.

SPINACH AND FETA STUFFED CHICKEN BREAST

COOK TIME: 35 MIN   SERVICE: 2 PERSONS

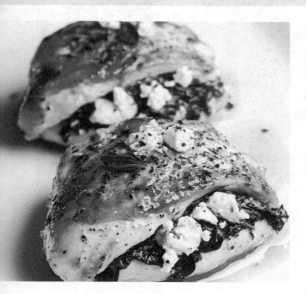

INGREDIENTS

- **2 boneless, skinless chicken breasts**
- **1 cup fresh spinach, chopped**
- **1/4 cup crumbled feta cheese**
- **1 clove garlic, minced**
- **1 tablespoon olive oil**
- **Salt and pepper to taste**
- **1/4 teaspoon dried oregano (optional)**
- **1 tablespoon lemon juice (for garnish)**

NUTRITIONAL INFORMATION (PER SERVING)

- Calories: 350 kcal
- Protein: 35g
- Fat: 20g
- Carbohydrates: 3g
- Fiber: 1g

INSTRUCTIONS

1. Preheat Oven: Preheat your oven to 375°F (190°C).
2. Prepare the Filling: In a small bowl, mix the chopped spinach, crumbled feta, minced garlic, olive oil, salt, pepper, and dried oregano.
3. Stuff the Chicken Breasts: Using a sharp knife, carefully cut a slit horizontally into the side of each chicken breast to create a pocket (be careful not to cut all the way through). Stuff the spinach and feta mixture evenly into each pocket. Secure the opening with toothpicks if needed.
4. Sear the Chicken: In an oven-safe skillet, heat a small amount of olive oil over medium heat. Sear the stuffed chicken breasts for 2-3 minutes on each side until golden brown.
5. Bake: Transfer the skillet to the preheated oven and bake the chicken breasts for 18-20 minutes, or until the internal temperature reaches 165°F (74°C).
6. Serve: Remove the chicken breasts from the oven and drizzle with lemon juice. Serve hot, and enjoy!

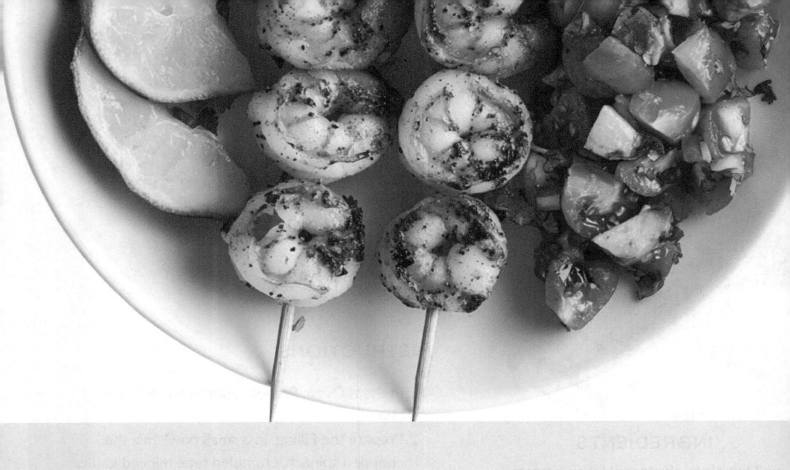

Dinner

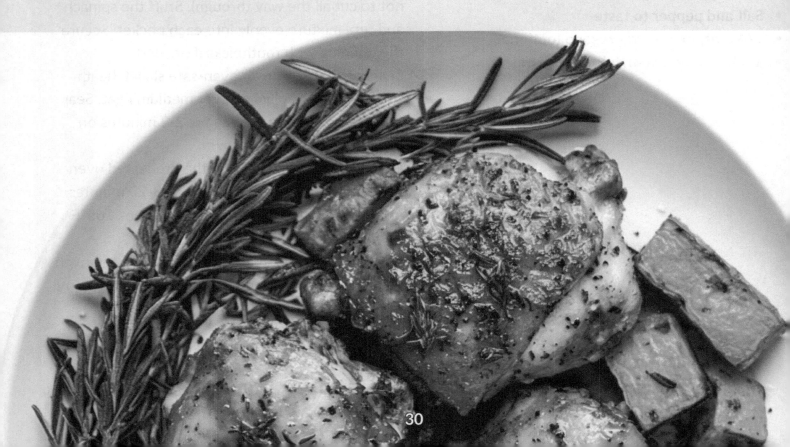

30

BAKED LEMON GARLIC SALMON

COOK TIME: **25 MIN**   SERVICE: **2 PERSONS**

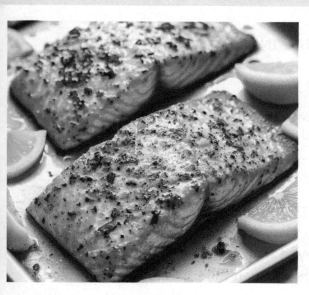

INGREDIENTS

- **2 salmon fillets (4-6 oz each)**
- **1 tablespoon olive oil**
- **2 garlic cloves, minced**
- **1 tablespoon fresh lemon juice**
- **1 teaspoon lemon zest**
- **Salt and pepper to taste**
- **1/2 teaspoon dried thyme (optional)**
- **Fresh parsley for garnish (optional)**
- **Lemon wedges for serving (optional)**

NUTRITIONAL INFORMATION (PER SERVING)

- Calories: 350 kcal
- Protein: 34g
- Fat: 22g
- Carbohydrates: 2g
- Fiber: 0g

INSTRUCTIONS

1. Preheat the Oven: Preheat your oven to 400°F (200°C).
2. Prepare the Salmon: Place the salmon fillets on a baking sheet lined with parchment paper or aluminum foil.
3. Make the Marinade: In a small bowl, mix the olive oil, minced garlic, lemon juice, lemon zest, salt, pepper, and thyme (if using).
4. Marinate the Salmon: Brush the marinade over the salmon fillets, ensuring they are evenly coated.
5. Bake the Salmon: Bake the salmon in the preheated oven for 12-15 minutes, or until the salmon flakes easily with a fork and reaches an internal temperature of 145°F (63°C).
6. Serve: Remove the salmon from the oven and garnish with fresh parsley and lemon wedges. Serve immediately with your favorite anti-inflammatory side dish, such as steamed broccoli or quinoa.

HERB-ROASTED CHICKEN THIGHS WITH SWEET POTATOES

COOK TIME: **50 MIN**   SERVICE: **2 PERSONS**

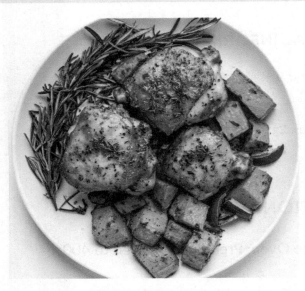

INGREDIENTS

- **2 bone-in, skin-on chicken thighs (about 6 oz each)**
- **2 medium sweet potatoes (about 8 oz each), cut into 1-inch cubes**
- **1 tbsp olive oil**
- **1 tbsp fresh rosemary, chopped (or 1 tsp dried rosemary)**
- **1 tbsp fresh thyme, chopped (or 1 tsp dried thyme)**
- **1 garlic clove, minced**
- **1/2 tsp paprika**
- **Salt and black pepper to taste**
- **1/2 lemon, for squeezing**
- **1/2 red onion, roughly chopped (optional)**

NUTRITIONAL INFORMATION (PER SERVING)

- Protein: 25g
- Fat: 15g
- Carbohydrates: 40g
- Calories: 450 kcal

INSTRUCTIONS

1. Preheat oven to 425°F (220°C).
2. Prepare the chicken thighs: Pat dry the chicken thighs with paper towels and season them with salt, pepper, paprika, rosemary, thyme, and garlic.
3. Toss the sweet potatoes: In a separate bowl, toss sweet potato cubes and red onion (optional) with olive oil, salt, pepper, and a bit of the rosemary and thyme.
4. Arrange on a baking sheet: Spread the sweet potatoes and onions on a baking sheet, and place the seasoned chicken thighs on top.
5. Roast: Place the sheet in the preheated oven and roast for 35-40 minutes, or until the chicken reaches an internal temperature of 165°F (75°C) and the sweet potatoes are tender and caramelized.
6. Finish with lemon: Once out of the oven, squeeze lemon juice over the chicken and vegetables for extra brightness.
7. Serve: Let the chicken rest for 5 minutes before serving with the roasted sweet potatoes.

CAULIFLOWER RICE STIR-FRY WITH SHRIMP

COOK TIME: **25 MIN**   SERVICE: **2 PERSONS**

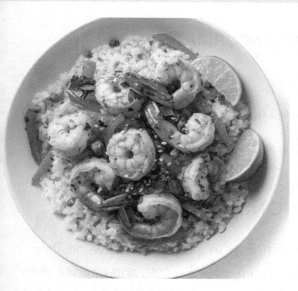

NUTRITIONAL INFORMATION (PER SERVING)

- Protein: 30g
- Fat: 14g
- Carbohydrates: 12g
- Fiber: 5g
- Calories: 290 kcal

INGREDIENTS

- **12 oz shrimp, peeled and deveined**
- **3 cups cauliflower rice (about 1 medium head of cauliflower, riced)**
- **1 tbsp olive oil or avocado oil**
- **1/2 red bell pepper, diced**
- **1/2 cup carrots, julienned or thinly sliced**
- **1/4 cup green onions, chopped**
- **2 garlic cloves, minced**
- **1 tbsp fresh ginger, grated**
- **2 tbsp low-sodium tamari or soy sauce**
- **1 tbsp sesame oil (optional, for flavor)**
- **1/4 tsp turmeric (anti-inflammatory boost)**
- **Salt and pepper to taste**
- **1 tbsp sesame seeds (optional)**
- **1/2 lime, for serving**

INSTRUCTIONS

1. Prep the cauliflower rice: If using a fresh cauliflower head, pulse the cauliflower florets in a food processor until it resembles rice grains. Set aside.
2. Cook the shrimp: Heat 1/2 tbsp of olive oil in a large skillet over medium heat. Add the shrimp, season with salt and pepper, and cook for 2-3 minutes per side until pink and opaque. Remove from the skillet and set aside.
3. Stir-fry the vegetables: In the same skillet, add the remaining 1/2 tbsp of oil. Stir in the garlic, ginger, red bell pepper, and carrots. Cook for about 3-4 minutes until slightly softened.
4. Add the cauliflower rice: Stir in the cauliflower rice, turmeric, and tamari or soy sauce. Cook for another 5-7 minutes, stirring frequently until the cauliflower rice is tender.
5. Combine and finish: Return the cooked shrimp to the skillet. Stir everything together, allowing the flavors to combine for about 2 more minutes. Drizzle with sesame oil (optional) and garnish with sesame seeds and green onions.
6. Serve: Squeeze lime juice over the stir-fry just before serving for added brightness.

GRILLED SHRIMP SKEWERS WITH AVOCADO SALSA

COOK TIME: 25 MIN   SERVICE: 2 PERSONS

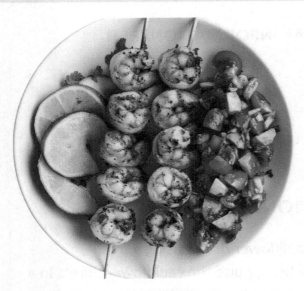

INGREDIENTS

For the Shrimp Skewers:
- **12 oz large shrimp, peeled and deveined**
- **1 tbsp olive oil**
- **1 tbsp lime juice**
- **1 garlic clove, minced**
- **1/2 tsp cumin**
- **1/4 tsp paprika**
- **Salt and black pepper to taste**
- **Wooden or metal skewers**

For the Avocado Salsa:
- **1 ripe avocado, diced**
- **1/2 small red onion, finely diced**
- **1/2 jalapeño, minced (optional)**
- **1/2 cup cherry tomatoes, halved**
- **1 tbsp fresh cilantro, chopped**
- **1 tbsp lime juice**
- **Salt and pepper to taste**

NUTRITIONAL INFORMATION (PER SERVING)

- Protein: 30g
- Fat: 22g
- Carbohydrates: 12g
- Fiber: 7g
- Calories: 350 kcal

INSTRUCTIONS

1. Prepare the shrimp: In a bowl, mix olive oil, lime juice, garlic, cumin, paprika, salt, and pepper. Add the shrimp, tossing to coat. Let marinate for 10-15 minutes while you prepare the salsa.
2. Make the avocado salsa: In a medium bowl, combine the diced avocado, red onion, jalapeño (if using), cherry tomatoes, cilantro, lime juice, salt, and pepper. Gently mix to combine and set aside.
3. Grill the shrimp: Preheat the grill (or grill pan) to medium-high heat. Thread the shrimp onto skewers (about 4-6 shrimp per skewer). Grill the shrimp for 2-3 minutes on each side until they are pink and opaque. Be careful not to overcook.
4. Serve: Place the grilled shrimp skewers on a plate and top with the avocado salsa. Serve immediately with an additional squeeze of lime juice if desired.

ZUCCHINI NOODLES WITH PESTO AND GRILLED CHICKEN

COOK TIME: **25 MIN**   SERVICE: **2 PERSONS**

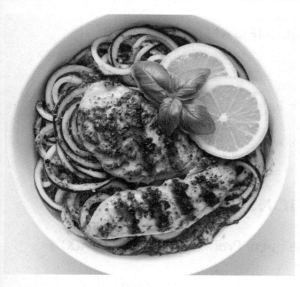

INGREDIENTS

For the Zucchini Noodles:
- 2 medium zucchinis, spiralized into noodles (about 3-4 cups)
- 1 tbsp olive oil
- Salt and pepper, to taste

For the Grilled Chicken:
- 2 boneless, skinless chicken breasts (about 6 oz each)
- 1 tbsp olive oil
- 1/2 tsp garlic powder
- 1/2 tsp paprika
- Salt and black pepper, to taste

For the Pesto:
- 1/2 cup fresh basil leaves
- 1/4 cup raw walnuts or pine nuts
- 1 garlic clove
- 2 tbsp olive oil
- 1 tbsp lemon juice
- 2 tbsp water, to thin (optional)
- Salt and pepper, to taste

NUTRITIONAL INFORMATION (PER SERVING)

- Protein: 32g
- Fat: 22g
- Carbohydrates: 8g
- Fiber: 3g
- Calories: 360 kcal

INSTRUCTIONS

1. Grill the chicken: Preheat the grill (or grill pan) to medium-high heat. Rub the chicken breasts with olive oil, garlic powder, paprika, salt, and pepper. Grill for 6-7 minutes on each side, or until the internal temperature reaches 165°F (75°C). Let the chicken rest for 5 minutes before slicing.
2. Make the pesto: While the chicken is grilling, prepare the pesto. In a food processor, combine basil, walnuts (or pine nuts), garlic, olive oil, lemon juice, and a pinch of salt and pepper. Blend until smooth. If needed, add a bit of water to reach the desired consistency. Set aside.
3. Cook the zucchini noodles: In a large skillet, heat 1 tbsp of olive oil over medium heat. Add the zucchini noodles and sauté for 2-3 minutes until just tender. Season with salt and pepper.
4. Combine and serve: Toss the zucchini noodles with the prepared pesto until evenly coated. Divide the noodles between two plates and top with the sliced grilled chicken. Optionally, garnish with additional basil or a sprinkle of nuts for extra flavor and crunch.

BAKED HALIBUT WITH LEMON AND ASPARAGUS

COOK TIME: **25 MIN**   SERVICE: **2 PERSONS**

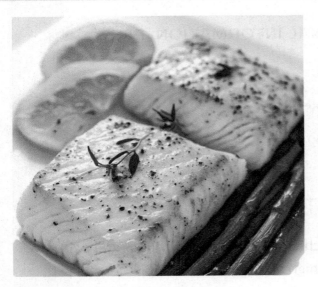

INGREDIENTS

- **2 halibut fillets (about 6 oz each)**
- **1 bunch asparagus (about 12 spears), trimmed**
- **2 tbsp olive oil**
- **1 lemon, thinly sliced**
- **2 garlic cloves, minced**
- **1/2 tsp dried thyme**
- **Salt and black pepper to taste**
- **1 tbsp fresh parsley, chopped (optional for garnish)**

NUTRITIONAL INFORMATION (PER SERVING)

- Protein: 35g
- Fat: 14g
- Carbohydrates: 8g
- Fiber: 4g
- Calories: 320 kcal

INSTRUCTIONS

1. Preheat the oven: Preheat your oven to 400°F (200°C).
2. Prepare the baking sheet: Line a baking sheet with parchment paper or lightly grease with olive oil.
3. Season the halibut: Place the halibut fillets on one side of the baking sheet. Drizzle with 1 tbsp of olive oil, then season with salt, pepper, thyme, and minced garlic. Place a few lemon slices on top of the halibut fillets.
4. Prepare the asparagus: On the other side of the baking sheet, arrange the asparagus spears. Drizzle the remaining 1 tbsp of olive oil over the asparagus and season with salt and pepper. Toss to coat.
5. Bake: Place the baking sheet in the oven and bake for 12-15 minutes, or until the halibut is opaque and flakes easily with a fork, and the asparagus is tender but still crisp.
6. Serve: Garnish the halibut with fresh parsley and serve with the roasted asparagus and a squeeze of fresh lemon juice.

MEDITERRANEAN BAKED COD WITH OLIVES AND TOMATOES

COOK TIME: 25 MIN   SERVICE: 2 PERSONS

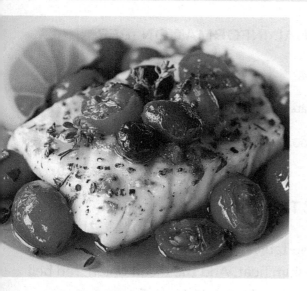

NUTRITIONAL INFORMATION (PER SERVING)

- Protein: 32g
- Fat: 12g
- Carbohydrates: 8g
- Fiber: 3g
- Calories: 280 kcal

INGREDIENTS

- 2 cod fillets (about 6 oz each)
- 1 cup cherry tomatoes, halved
- 1/4 cup Kalamata olives, pitted and halved
- 2 garlic cloves, minced
- 1 tbsp olive oil
- 1/2 tsp dried oregano
- 1/2 tsp dried thyme
- Salt and black pepper, to taste
- 1/2 lemon, sliced
- 1 tbsp fresh parsley, chopped (for garnish)

INSTRUCTIONS

1. Preheat oven: Preheat your oven to 400°F (200°C).
2. Prepare the baking dish: In a small baking dish, place the cod fillets. Season both sides with salt, pepper, oregano, and thyme. Drizzle 1 tbsp of olive oil over the fillets.
3. Add the vegetables: Surround the cod with cherry tomatoes, Kalamata olives, and minced garlic. Lay lemon slices on top of the cod fillets for flavor.
4. Bake: Place the baking dish in the oven and bake for 12-15 minutes, or until the cod is opaque and flakes easily with a fork.
5. Garnish and serve: Remove from the oven and sprinkle fresh parsley on top before serving. Serve the cod with the baked tomatoes and olives on the side.

TURKEY CHILI

COOK TIME: **40 MIN**   SERVICE: **2 PERSONS**

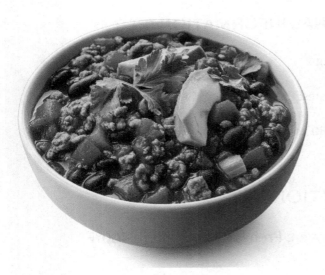

NUTRITIONAL INFORMATION (PER SERVING)

- Protein: 28g
- Fat: 14g
- Carbohydrates: 30g
- Fiber: 10g
- Calories: 360 kcal

INGREDIENTS

- 8 oz ground turkey (lean)
- 1/2 small onion, diced
- 1/2 red bell pepper, diced
- 2 garlic cloves, minced
- 1/2 cup diced tomatoes (canned, no salt added)
- 1/2 cup black beans (canned, drained and rinsed)
- 1/2 cup kidney beans (canned, drained and rinsed)
- 1 tbsp olive oil
- 1 tsp chili powder
- 1/2 tsp ground cumin
- 1/2 tsp smoked paprika
- 1/4 tsp ground turmeric (for anti-inflammatory benefits)
- Salt and black pepper to taste
- 1/2 cup low-sodium chicken broth
- 1/2 avocado, diced (for garnish)
- 1 tbsp fresh cilantro, chopped (for garnish)

INSTRUCTIONS

1. Sauté vegetables: In a medium pot, heat olive oil over medium heat. Add the diced onion, red bell pepper, and garlic. Sauté for 4-5 minutes until softened.
2. Brown the turkey: Add the ground turkey to the pot. Cook for about 5-7 minutes, breaking it up with a spoon, until browned and cooked through.
3. Add seasonings: Stir in the chili powder, cumin, smoked paprika, turmeric, salt, and pepper. Cook for 1-2 minutes until fragrant.
4. Add tomatoes and beans: Pour in the diced tomatoes, black beans, kidney beans, and chicken broth. Stir everything together.
5. Simmer: Bring the chili to a boil, then reduce the heat to low. Simmer uncovered for 20 minutes, stirring occasionally, to allow the flavors to meld and the chili to thicken.
6. Serve: Once done, divide the chili between two bowls. Garnish with diced avocado and fresh cilantro for an extra anti-inflammatory boost.

SPAGHETTI SQUASH WITH MARINARA AND TURKEY MEATBALLS

COOK TIME: 50 MIN   SERVICE: 2 PERSONS

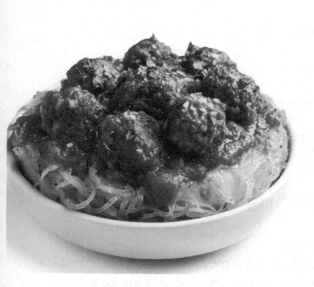

INGREDIENTS

For the Spaghetti Squash:
- 1 medium spaghetti squash (about 2 lbs)
- 1 tbsp olive oil
- Salt and black pepper to taste

For the Turkey Meatballs:
- 8 oz ground turkey (lean)
- 1 garlic clove, minced
- 1/4 cup onion, finely diced
- 1 tbsp fresh parsley, chopped (or 1 tsp dried parsley)
- 1/4 tsp dried oregano
- 1/4 tsp ground turmeric (for anti-inflammatory benefits)
- 1/4 tsp black pepper
- Salt to taste
- 1 tbsp olive oil (for cooking the meatballs)

For the Marinara Sauce:
- 1 cup marinara sauce (low-sodium, store-bought, or homemade)
- 1 tbsp olive oil
- 1 garlic clove, minced
- 1/4 tsp red pepper flakes (optional for heat)
- 1 tbsp fresh basil, chopped (optional)

NUTRITIONAL INFORMATION (PER SERVING)

- Protein: 28g
- Fat: 18g
- Carbohydrates: 26g
- Fiber: 6g
- Calories: 390 kcal

INSTRUCTIONS

Prepare the Spaghetti Squash:
1. Preheat oven: Preheat your oven to 400°F (200°C).
2. Roast the squash: Cut the spaghetti squash in half lengthwise and scoop out the seeds. Drizzle each half with olive oil, then season with salt and pepper. Place the squash cut-side down on a baking sheet lined with parchment paper. Roast for 35-40 minutes, or until the flesh is tender and easily shredded with a fork.
3. Shred the squash: Once done, use a fork to scrape out the strands of the spaghetti squash, creating "noodles."

Make the Turkey Meatballs:
1. Mix the meatball ingredients: In a bowl, combine the ground turkey, minced garlic, onion, parsley, oregano, turmeric, black pepper, and salt. Form the mixture into small meatballs, about 1-1.5 inches in diameter.
2. Cook the meatballs: Heat 1 tbsp of olive oil in a skillet over medium heat. Add the meatballs and cook for 8-10 minutes, turning occasionally until browned and cooked through.

Prepare the Marinara Sauce:
1. Heat the sauce: In a small saucepan, heat 1 tbsp olive oil over medium heat. Add the minced garlic and red pepper flakes (if using) and sauté for 1 minute. Add the marinara sauce and simmer for 5-7 minutes until heated through. Stir in fresh basil, if desired.

Serve:
1. Assemble the dish: Divide the spaghetti squash noodles between two plates. Top with the marinara sauce and place the turkey meatballs on top. Garnish with extra fresh basil or parsley if desired.

GRILLED CHICKEN WITH QUINOA AND ROASTED VEGETABLES

COOK TIME: 40 MIN   SERVICE: 2 PERSONS

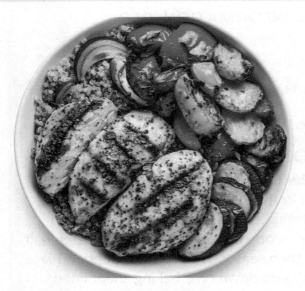

INGREDIENTS

For the Grilled Chicken:
- 2 boneless, skinless chicken breasts (about 6 oz each)
- 1 tbsp olive oil
- 1 garlic clove, minced
- 1 tsp dried oregano
- 1/2 tsp ground turmeric (for anti-inflammatory benefits)
- 1/2 tsp paprika
- Salt and black pepper to taste
- Juice of 1/2 lemon

For the Quinoa:
- 1/2 cup quinoa, rinsed
- 1 cup low-sodium chicken or vegetable broth (or water)
- 1/2 tbsp olive oil
- 1 tbsp fresh parsley, chopped (for garnish)

For the Roasted Vegetables:
- 1 medium zucchini, sliced
- 1 red bell pepper, sliced
- 1/2 red onion, sliced
- 1 tbsp olive oil
- 1/2 tsp dried thyme
- Salt and black pepper to taste

NUTRITIONAL INFORMATION (PER SERVING)

- Protein: 35g
- Fat: 18g
- Carbohydrates: 28g
- Fiber: 5g
- Calories: 430 kcal

INSTRUCTIONS

Prepare the Quinoa:
1. Cook the quinoa: In a medium saucepan, combine quinoa and broth (or water) and bring to a boil. Reduce the heat to low, cover, and simmer for 15 minutes, or until the quinoa is cooked and the liquid is absorbed. Fluff with a fork and drizzle with olive oil. Garnish with fresh parsley.

Grill the Chicken:
1. Marinate the chicken: In a small bowl, mix olive oil, garlic, oregano, turmeric, paprika, salt, pepper, and lemon juice. Rub the marinade onto the chicken breasts and let sit for 10-15 minutes.
2. Grill the chicken: Preheat a grill or grill pan to medium-high heat. Grill the chicken for 6-7 minutes per side, or until the internal temperature reaches 165°F (75°C). Remove from heat and let rest for 5 minutes before slicing.

Roast the Vegetables:
1. Preheat oven: Preheat your oven to 400°F (200°C).
2. Roast the vegetables: Toss the zucchini, red bell pepper, and red onion with olive oil, thyme, salt, and pepper. Spread the vegetables on a baking sheet and roast for 20-25 minutes, or until tender and lightly browned.

Assemble the Dish:
1. Serve: Divide the cooked quinoa between two plates. Top with sliced grilled chicken and roasted vegetables. Optionally, garnish with additional fresh parsley or a squeeze of lemon juice.

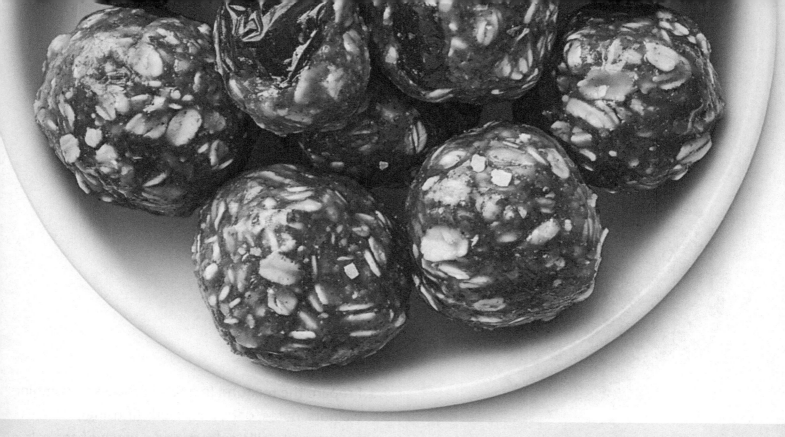

Snack and Appetizer

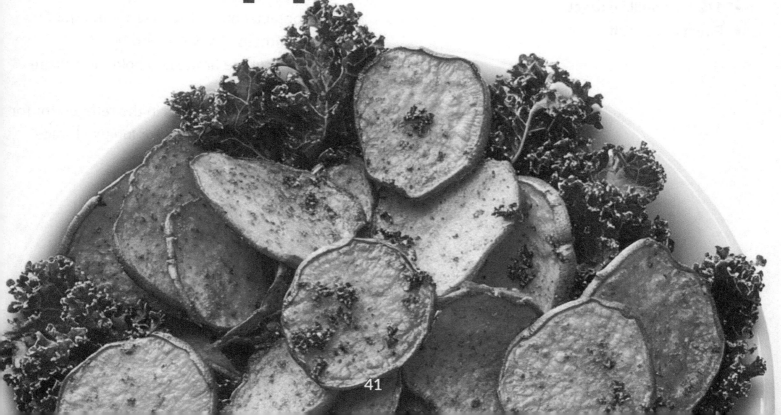

WALNUT AND DATE ENERGY BITES

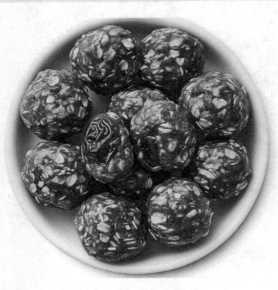

INGREDIENTS

- **1/2 cup walnuts**
- **1/4 cup dates, pitted**
- **1/8 cup oats (gluten-free, if needed)**
- **1 tbsp chia seeds (optional, for extra fiber and omega-3s)**
- **1/2 tsp ground cinnamon**
- **1/2 tsp vanilla extract**
- **Pinch of sea salt**

NUTRITIONAL INFORMATION (PER SERVING)

- Protein: 5g
- Fat: 11g
- Carbohydrates: 18g
- Fiber: 4g
- Calories: 200 kcal

INSTRUCTIONS

1. Prepare the mixture: In a food processor, combine walnuts, dates, oats, chia seeds (if using), cinnamon, vanilla extract, and a pinch of sea salt. Pulse until the mixture forms a sticky, cohesive dough.
2. Form the bites: Scoop out about 1 tablespoon of the mixture at a time and roll it into bite-sized balls with your hands. You should get around 8-10 energy bites from this recipe.
3. Chill: Place the energy bites on a plate or in an airtight container and refrigerate for at least 30 minutes to firm up. They can also be eaten immediately but are firmer and hold their shape better when chilled.
4. Store: Keep the energy bites in the refrigerator for up to 1 week or freeze them for longer storage.

COTTAGE CHEESE WITH PINEAPPLE AND FLAXSEEDS

COOK TIME: **5 MIN**   SERVICE: **2 PERSONS**

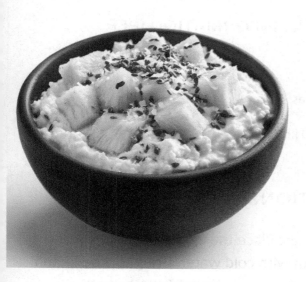

INGREDIENTS

- **1 cup low-fat cottage cheese (about 8 oz)**
- **1/2 cup fresh pineapple, diced**
- **1 tbsp ground flaxseeds**
- **1 tsp honey (optional, for extra sweetness)**
- **1 tbsp unsweetened shredded coconut (optional, for texture)**

NUTRITIONAL INFORMATION (PER SERVING)

- Protein: 12g
- Fat: 6g
- Carbohydrates: 16g
- Fiber: 3g
- Calories: 180 kcal

INSTRUCTIONS

1. Prepare the ingredients: In two serving bowls, divide the cottage cheese evenly (1/2 cup per bowl).
2. Top with pineapple: Divide the diced pineapple between the two bowls, placing it on top of the cottage cheese.
3. Add flaxseeds: Sprinkle 1/2 tbsp of ground flaxseeds over each bowl for added fiber and omega-3 fatty acids.
4. Optional toppings: Drizzle each bowl with 1/2 tsp honey for sweetness and sprinkle a bit of shredded coconut for extra texture, if desired.
5. Serve immediately: Enjoy this refreshing snack or appetizer chilled.

DEVILED EGGS WITH AVOCADO

COOK TIME: **20 MIN**   SERVICE: **2 PERSONS**

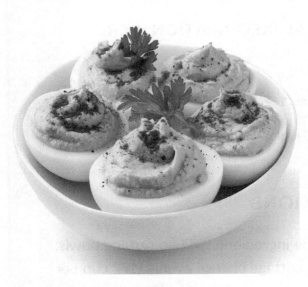

INGREDIENTS

- **4 large eggs**
- **1/2 ripe avocado**
- **1 tsp Dijon mustard**
- **1 tsp lemon juice**
- **1/8 tsp garlic powder**
- **Salt and black pepper, to taste**
- **Paprika (for garnish)**
- **Chopped fresh parsley (optional, for garnish)**

NUTRITIONAL INFORMATION (PER SERVING)

- Protein: 12g
- Fat: 14g
- Carbohydrates: 4g
- Fiber: 3g
- Calories: 190 kcal

INSTRUCTIONS

1. Boil the eggs: Place the eggs in a saucepan and cover them with cold water. Bring to a boil, then reduce the heat and simmer for 10 minutes. Remove from heat and transfer the eggs to an ice bath to cool for 5 minutes.
2. Peel and halve the eggs: Once the eggs are cool, peel them and cut them in half lengthwise. Carefully scoop out the yolks and place them in a bowl.
3. Prepare the filling: Mash the avocado with a fork in the bowl with the egg yolks. Add the Dijon mustard, lemon juice, garlic powder, salt, and black pepper. Mix until smooth and creamy.
4. Stuff the eggs: Spoon the avocado mixture back into the egg whites, filling the hollow center of each half.
5. Garnish: Sprinkle the deviled eggs with paprika and chopped parsley for garnish, if desired.
6. Serve immediately: Enjoy as a snack or appetizer. These deviled eggs can also be refrigerated for up to 1 day.

CHICKPEA SALAD LETTUCE WRAPS

COOK TIME: **10 MIN**   SERVICE: **2 PERSONS**

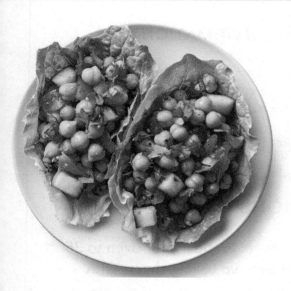

INGREDIENTS

- **1 cup canned chickpeas (drained and rinsed)**
- **1 tbsp olive oil**
- **1 tbsp lemon juice**
- **1/4 tsp ground turmeric (for anti-inflammatory benefits)**
- **1/4 tsp ground cumin**
- **1/2 garlic clove, minced**
- **1 tbsp fresh parsley, chopped**
- **Salt and black pepper, to taste**
- **4 large romaine or butter lettuce leaves (for wrapping)**
- **1/4 cup diced cucumber (optional for crunch)**
- **1/4 cup diced tomato (optional for extra flavor)**

NUTRITIONAL INFORMATION (PER SERVING)

- Protein: 6g
- Fat: 7g
- Carbohydrates: 16g
- Fiber: 5g
- Calories: 160 kcal

INSTRUCTIONS

1. Prepare the chickpea salad: In a bowl, mash the chickpeas with a fork or potato masher, leaving some texture (don't mash them completely smooth). Add olive oil, lemon juice, turmeric, cumin, minced garlic, and parsley. Stir until well combined. Season with salt and pepper to taste.
2. Assemble the lettuce wraps: Lay out the lettuce leaves. Spoon the chickpea mixture into the center of each leaf.
3. Optional toppings: If desired, top the chickpea salad with diced cucumber and tomato for added crunch and flavor.
4. Serve immediately: Fold the lettuce around the chickpea salad and enjoy as a light, anti-inflammatory snack or appetizer.

SWEET POTATO AND KALE CHIPS

COOK TIME: 35 MIN   SERVICE: 2 PERSONS

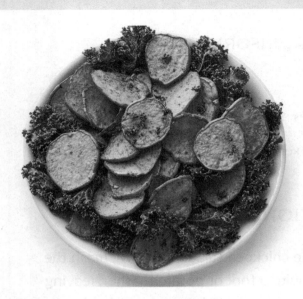

INGREDIENTS

For the Sweet Potato Chips:

- 1 medium sweet potato (about 6 oz), thinly sliced (1/8 inch thick)
- 1 tbsp olive oil
- 1/4 tsp ground turmeric (optional, for anti-inflammatory benefits)
- Salt and pepper, to taste

For the Kale Chips:

- 2 cups kale leaves, stems removed, torn into bite-sized pieces
- 1 tbsp olive oil
- 1/4 tsp garlic powder
- Salt, to taste

NUTRITIONAL INFORMATION (PER SERVING)

- Protein: 3g
- Fat: 10g
- Carbohydrates: 22g
- Fiber: 4g
- Calories: 180 kcal

INSTRUCTIONS

1. Preheat the oven: Preheat your oven to 350°F (175°C) and line two baking sheets with parchment paper.

For the Sweet Potato Chips:

1. Prepare the sweet potatoes: In a bowl, toss the thinly sliced sweet potatoes with 1 tbsp olive oil, turmeric (if using), salt, and pepper until evenly coated.
2. Bake the sweet potatoes: Arrange the sweet potato slices in a single layer on one of the prepared baking sheets. Bake for 20-25 minutes, flipping halfway through, until the edges are crispy and the centers are tender. Keep an eye on them to prevent burning.

For the Kale Chips:

1. Prepare the kale: In a separate bowl, toss the kale leaves with 1 tbsp olive oil, garlic powder, and a pinch of salt until evenly coated.
2. Bake the kale: Spread the kale leaves in a single layer on the second baking sheet. Bake for 10-12 minutes, until the edges are crispy and the kale is lightly browned. Check after 10 minutes to avoid overcooking.
3. Serve: Once both the sweet potato and kale chips are done, let them cool slightly and serve them together as a healthy, anti-inflammatory snack.

ROASTED RED PEPPER HUMMUS WITH VEGGIE STICKS

COOK TIME: **10** MIN   SERVICE: **2 PERSONS**

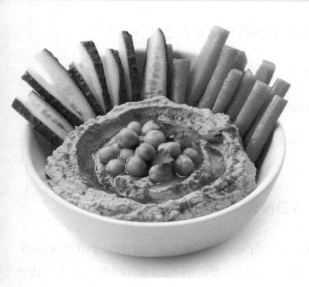

INGREDIENTS

For the Hummus:
- 1/2 cup canned chickpeas (drained and rinsed)
- 1/4 cup roasted red bell peppers (jarred or homemade)
- 1 tbsp tahini (sesame seed paste)
- 1 tbsp olive oil
- 1 tbsp lemon juice
- 1/2 garlic clove, minced
- 1/4 tsp ground cumin
- Salt and black pepper, to taste
- 1-2 tbsp water (to thin, if necessary)

For the Veggie Sticks:
- 1 small cucumber, sliced into sticks
- 1 carrot, sliced into sticks
- 1 small bell pepper (any color), sliced into sticks

NUTRITIONAL INFORMATION (PER SERVING)

- Protein: 5g
- Fat: 10g
- Carbohydrates: 19g
- Fiber: 6g
- Calories: 210 kcal

INSTRUCTIONS

1. Prepare the hummus: In a food processor, combine chickpeas, roasted red peppers, tahini, olive oil, lemon juice, garlic, cumin, salt, and pepper. Blend until smooth and creamy. Add 1-2 tbsp of water as needed to achieve your desired consistency.
2. Prepare the veggie sticks: While the hummus is blending, cut the cucumber, carrot, and bell pepper into sticks for dipping.
3. Serve: Spoon the hummus into a serving dish and enjoy with the fresh veggie sticks on the side.

SARDINES ON WHOLE GRAIN CRACKERS

COOK TIME: **5 MIN**   SERVICE: **2 PERSONS**

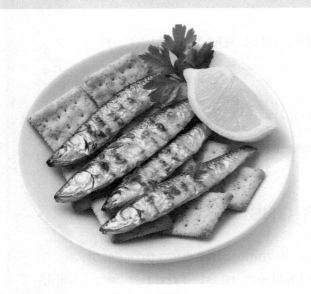

INGREDIENTS

- **1 can sardines (packed in olive oil, about 3.75 oz)**
- **8 whole-grain crackers**
- **1 tbsp lemon juice**
- **1 tsp Dijon mustard**
- **1 tsp olive oil (optional, if sardines are in water)**
- **1 tbsp fresh parsley, chopped (optional for garnish)**
- **Salt and black pepper, to taste**

NUTRITIONAL INFORMATION (PER SERVING)

- Protein: 13g
- Fat: 11g
- Carbohydrates: 16g
- Fiber: 3g
- Calories: 220 kcal

INSTRUCTIONS

1. Prepare the sardines: Drain the sardines (if packed in water) and transfer them to a small bowl. If they are packed in olive oil, you can use the oil for additional flavor or drizzle 1 tsp of fresh olive oil if desired.
2. Mix the flavoring: Add lemon juice, Dijon mustard, salt, and pepper to the sardines. Lightly mash and mix everything together, but keep some texture intact.
3. Assemble the crackers: Lay out the whole-grain crackers and spoon the sardine mixture evenly onto each cracker.
4. Garnish: Optionally, sprinkle with fresh parsley for an extra burst of freshness and flavor.
5. Serve: Enjoy immediately as a quick, nutritious snack or appetizer.

FROZEN GRAPES WITH ALMOND BUTTER

COOK TIME: 2-3 HOURS (INCLUDING FREEZING)
SERVICE: 2 PERSONS

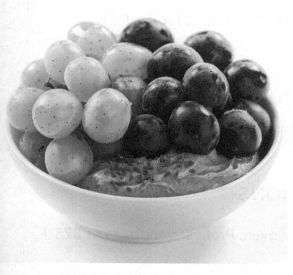

INGREDIENTS

- **1 cup seedless grapes (red or green)**
- **2 tbsp almond butter (unsweetened)**
- **1 tsp ground cinnamon (optional, for extra flavor)**
- **1 tsp chia seeds (optional, for added fiber and omega-3s)**

NUTRITIONAL INFORMATION (PER SERVING)

- Protein: 4g
- Fat: 9g
- Carbohydrates: 18g
- Fiber: 4g
- Calories: 160 kcal

INSTRUCTIONS

1. Freeze the grapes: Wash the grapes and spread them out in a single layer on a baking sheet. Place the baking sheet in the freezer for at least 2-3 hours, or until the grapes are fully frozen.
2. Prepare the almond butter: In a small bowl, stir the almond butter to ensure it is smooth and creamy. You can optionally mix in ground cinnamon for added flavor.
3. Serve: Once the grapes are frozen, divide them between two bowls. Serve with a small dish of almond butter for dipping. Optionally, sprinkle chia seeds on top for extra texture and nutrition.
4. Enjoy immediately: Frozen grapes paired with creamy almond butter make for a refreshing, nutrient-packed snack.

MINI BELL PEPPER "NACHOS"

COOK TIME: **20 MIN**   SERVICE: **2 PERSONS**

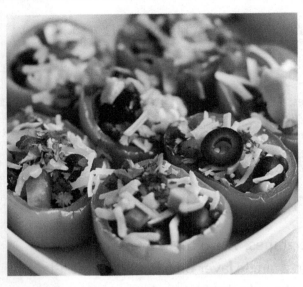

INGREDIENTS

- 6 mini bell peppers, halved and seeds removed
- 1/2 cup black beans, drained and rinsed
- 1/4 cup shredded cheese (cheddar, Monterey Jack, or dairy-free alternative)
- 1/4 cup diced tomatoes
- 1 tbsp sliced black olives (optional)
- 1 tbsp fresh cilantro, chopped
- 1/2 tsp ground cumin
- 1/4 tsp paprika
- Salt and pepper, to taste
- 1/2 avocado, diced (optional, for topping)
- 1 tbsp Greek yogurt or dairy-free yogurt (optional, for topping)

NUTRITIONAL INFORMATION (PER SERVING)

- Protein: 10g
- Fat: 11g
- Carbohydrates: 19g
- Fiber: 7g
- Calories: 210 kcal

INSTRUCTIONS

1. Preheat the oven: Preheat your oven to 375°F (190°C).
2. Prepare the bell peppers: Slice the mini bell peppers in half lengthwise and remove the seeds. Place them cut-side up on a baking sheet lined with parchment paper.
3. Season the beans: In a small bowl, mix the black beans with cumin, paprika, salt, and pepper.
4. Assemble the nachos: Spoon the seasoned black beans evenly into the bell pepper halves. Top with shredded cheese and diced tomatoes. Optionally, add sliced black olives for extra flavor.
5. Bake: Place the baking sheet in the oven and bake for 10-12 minutes, or until the cheese is melted and the peppers are slightly tender.
6. Add toppings: Remove the peppers from the oven and garnish with fresh cilantro, diced avocado, and a dollop of Greek yogurt (if using).
7. Serve immediately: Enjoy these colorful, healthy "nachos" as a fun, anti-inflammatory snack or appetizer.

ZUCCHINI FRIES

COOK TIME: 30 MIN   **SERVICE: 2 PERSONS**

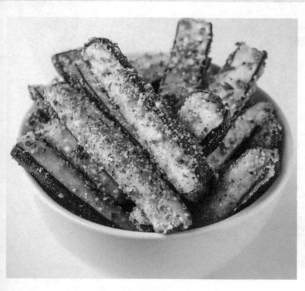

INGREDIENTS

- **1 medium zucchini**
- **1 tbsp olive oil**
- **1/4 cup almond flour (or breadcrumbs if preferred)**
- **1/4 cup grated Parmesan cheese (optional for extra flavor)**
- **1/2 tsp garlic powder**
- **1/2 tsp paprika**
- **Salt and black pepper, to taste**
- **1/4 tsp turmeric (optional, for anti-inflammatory benefits)**

NUTRITIONAL INFORMATION (PER SERVING)

- Protein: 5g
- Fat: 10g
- Carbohydrates: 8g
- Fiber: 3g
- Calories: 140 kcal

INSTRUCTIONS

1. Preheat the oven: Preheat your oven to 400°F (200°C) and line a baking sheet with parchment paper.
2. Prepare the zucchini: Cut the zucchini into thin strips, about the size of traditional fries.
3. Season the fries: In a small bowl, combine almond flour, Parmesan cheese (if using), garlic powder, paprika, salt, pepper, and turmeric.
4. Coat the zucchini: Toss the zucchini strips in olive oil to coat them. Then, dredge each strip in the almond flour mixture, making sure each piece is coated evenly.
5. Bake: Arrange the zucchini fries in a single layer on the prepared baking sheet. Bake for 15-18 minutes, flipping halfway through, until golden brown and crispy.
6. Serve: Let the fries cool slightly and enjoy as a crunchy, anti-inflammatory snack or appetizer. They can be served with a yogurt-based dipping sauce or your favorite condiment.

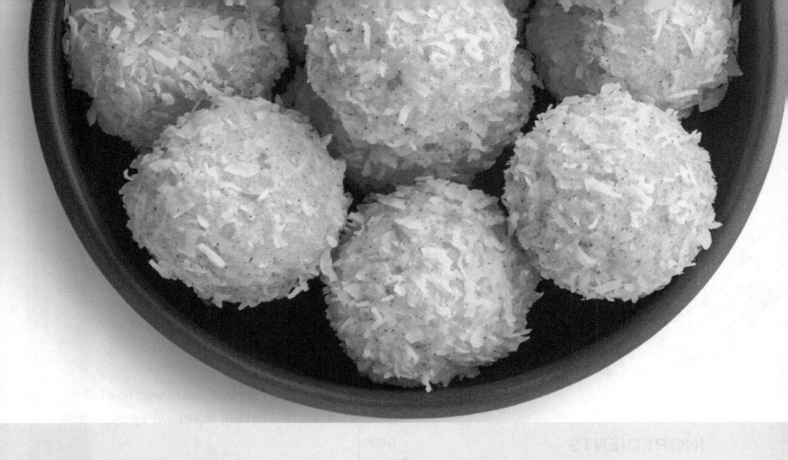

Dessert

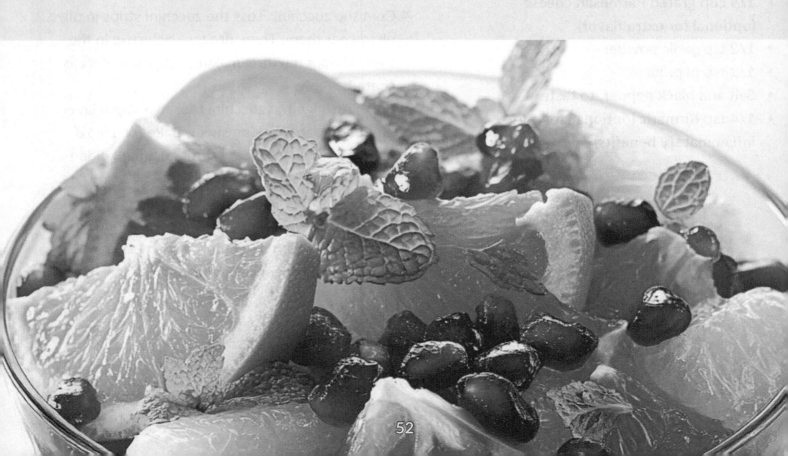

TURMERIC AND GINGER COCONUT MACAROONS

COOK TIME: 25 MIN   SERVICE: 2 PERSONS

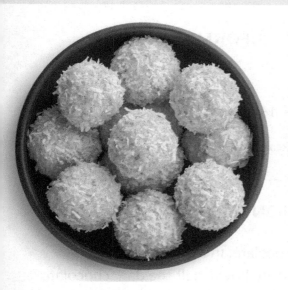

INGREDIENTS

- **1 cup shredded unsweetened coconut**
- **1 tbsp ground turmeric**
- **1/2 tsp ground ginger**
- **2 tbsp honey (or maple syrup)**
- **2 egg whites**
- **1/4 tsp vanilla extract (optional)**
- **Pinch of sea salt**

NUTRITIONAL INFORMATION (PER SERVING)

- Protein: 4g
- Fat: 14g
- Carbohydrates: 16g
- Fiber: 4g
- Calories: 210 kcal

INSTRUCTIONS

1. Preheat the oven: Preheat your oven to 325°F (160°C) and line a baking sheet with parchment paper.
2. Mix the ingredients: In a medium bowl, combine shredded coconut, turmeric, ginger, and a pinch of sea salt. In a separate bowl, whisk the egg whites until frothy. Gently fold the egg whites, honey, and vanilla extract (if using) into the coconut mixture.
3. Form the macaroons: Using a tablespoon, scoop small mounds of the mixture onto the prepared baking sheet. Press them lightly to form compact mounds.
4. Bake: Bake for 12-15 minutes, or until the tops are golden brown.
5. Cool: Remove the macaroons from the oven and allow them to cool on the baking sheet for a few minutes before transferring to a wire rack to cool completely.
6. Serve: Enjoy as a healthy, anti-inflammatory dessert or snack.

DARK CHOCOLATE-COVERED ALMONDS

COOK TIME: 25 MIN   SERVICE: 2 PERSONS

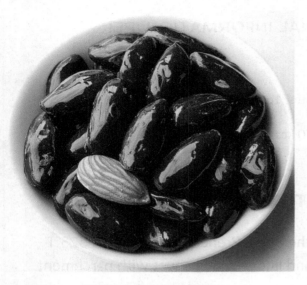

INGREDIENTS

- **1/2 cup raw almonds**
- **1/2 cup dark chocolate (70% cacao or higher)**
- **1/2 tsp coconut oil (optional, for smoother melting)**
- **1/4 tsp sea salt (optional, for sprinkling)**

NUTRITIONAL INFORMATION (PER SERVING)

- Protein: 6g
- Fat: 18g
- Carbohydrates: 16g
- Fiber: 6g
- Calories: 230 kcal

INSTRUCTIONS

1. Melt the chocolate: In a double boiler or a microwave-safe bowl, melt the dark chocolate with the coconut oil (if using) in 30-second intervals, stirring in between until fully melted and smooth.
2. Coat the almonds: Stir the raw almonds into the melted chocolate, making sure each almond is fully coated with chocolate.
3. Set the almonds: Using a fork or a small spoon, lift the chocolate-covered almonds one at a time and place them on a baking sheet lined with parchment paper.
4. Add sea salt: Lightly sprinkle the sea salt over the almonds while the chocolate is still soft, if desired.
5. Chill: Place the baking sheet in the refrigerator for 20-30 minutes, or until the chocolate is fully set.
6. Serve: Once the chocolate has hardened, enjoy the almonds as a satisfying, anti-inflammatory snack or dessert. Store any leftovers in an airtight container in the refrigerator.

FROZEN BANANA BITES WITH PEANUT BUTTER

COOK TIME: FREEZING TIME 90 MIN   SERVICE: 2 PERSONS

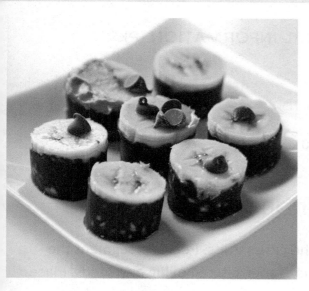

INGREDIENTS

- 1 large banana, sliced into 1/2-inch rounds
- 2 tbsp peanut butter (natural, unsweetened)
- 1/4 cup dark chocolate chips (70% cacao or higher)
- 1/2 tsp coconut oil (optional, for smoother melting)
- Pinch of sea salt (optional, for sprinkling)

NUTRITIONAL INFORMATION (PER SERVING)

- Protein: 6g
- Fat: 14g
- Carbohydrates: 26g
- Fiber: 4g
- Calories: 240 kcal

INSTRUCTIONS

1. Prepare the banana slices: Slice the banana into 1/2-inch rounds. Spread a small amount of peanut butter on half of the banana slices and top them with the remaining banana slices to form small "sandwiches."
2. Freeze the banana bites: Place the banana sandwiches on a parchment-lined baking sheet and freeze for about 1 hour until firm.
3. Melt the chocolate: In a microwave-safe bowl or double boiler, melt the dark chocolate chips with the coconut oil (if using) in 30-second intervals, stirring in between until smooth.
4. Dip the banana bites: Remove the frozen banana bites from the freezer. Dip each banana sandwich halfway into the melted chocolate and return them to the baking sheet. Optionally, sprinkle with a pinch of sea salt.
5. Set the chocolate: Place the baking sheet back in the freezer for another 15-20 minutes or until the chocolate is fully set.
6. Serve: Once the chocolate has hardened, enjoy the frozen banana bites as a cool, anti-inflammatory treat. Store any leftovers in an airtight container in the freezer.

CHILLED CITRUS FRUIT SALAD WITH MINT

COOK TIME: **10 MIN (CHILL TIME 30 MIN)**   SERVICE: **2 PERSONS**

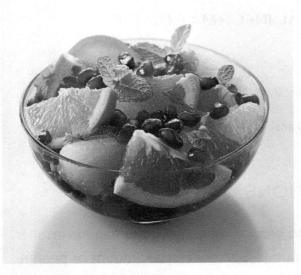

INGREDIENTS

- **1 orange, peeled and segmented**
- **1 grapefruit, peeled and segmented**
- **1/2 cup pomegranate seeds**
- **1 tbsp fresh mint, chopped**
- **1 tsp honey (optional, for added sweetness)**
- **1 tsp lime juice (optional, for extra tang)**

NUTRITIONAL INFORMATION (PER SERVING)

- Protein: 2g
- Fat: 1g
- Carbohydrates: 26g
- Fiber: 6g
- Calories: 130 kcal

INSTRUCTIONS

1. Prepare the citrus fruits: Peel and segment the orange and grapefruit, removing any seeds. Place the segments in a bowl.
2. Add the pomegranate seeds: Sprinkle the pomegranate seeds over the citrus segments.
3. Add mint and flavorings: Sprinkle the chopped fresh mint over the fruit. Optionally, drizzle honey and lime juice over the salad for added sweetness and tang.
4. Chill the salad: Cover the bowl and refrigerate the salad for 30 minutes to allow the flavors to meld and to serve it chilled.
5. Serve: Once chilled, divide the citrus fruit salad into two bowls and enjoy as a refreshing, anti-inflammatory dessert or snack.

DARK CHOCOLATE AVOCADO TRUFFLES

COOK TIME: **10 MIN (CHILL TIME 30 MIN)**   SERVICE: **2 PERSONS**

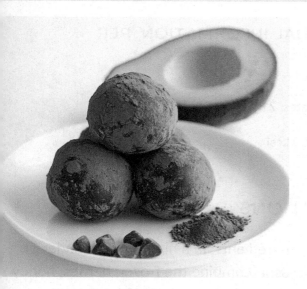

NUTRITIONAL INFORMATION (PER SERVING)

- Protein: 3g
- Fat: 15g
- Carbohydrates: 16g
- Fiber: 6g
- Calories: 200 kcal

INGREDIENTS

- **1 ripe avocado**
- **1/2 cup dark chocolate chips (70% cacao or higher)**
- **1/2 tsp vanilla extract (optional)**
- **2 tbsp unsweetened cocoa powder (for coating)**
- **1 tbsp honey or maple syrup (optional, for sweetness)**
-

INSTRUCTIONS

1. Melt the chocolate: In a microwave-safe bowl or using a double boiler, melt the dark chocolate chips until smooth. Stir every 30 seconds if microwaving to avoid burning.
2. Prepare the avocado: In a medium bowl, mash the ripe avocado until smooth and creamy, ensuring no lumps remain.
3. Mix the ingredients: Stir the melted chocolate into the mashed avocado, along with the vanilla extract and honey or maple syrup (if using). Mix until well combined.
4. Chill the mixture: Cover the mixture and refrigerate for 30-40 minutes, or until firm enough to handle.
5. Form the truffles: Once chilled, scoop out small portions of the mixture (about 1 tablespoon each) and roll them into balls with your hands.
6. Coat the truffles: Roll each truffle in unsweetened cocoa powder to coat evenly.
7. Serve: Enjoy immediately or refrigerate the truffles for an additional 10-15 minutes to firm up more before serving.

BERRY SORBET

COOK TIME: **10 MIN (FREEZE TIME 120 MIN)**   SERVICE: **2 PERSONS**

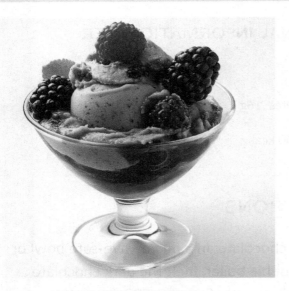

INGREDIENTS

- **2 cups mixed frozen berries (blueberries, raspberries, strawberries, or blackberries)**
- **1 tbsp honey or maple syrup (optional, for sweetness)**
- **1 tbsp fresh lemon juice**
- **1/4 cup water (or more if needed)**

NUTRITIONAL INFORMATION (PER SERVING)

- Protein: 1g
- Fat: 0g
- Carbohydrates: 21g
- Fiber: 6g
- Calories: 100 kcal

INSTRUCTIONS

1. Blend the ingredients: In a high-speed blender or food processor, combine the frozen berries, honey (if using), lemon juice, and water. Blend until smooth, scraping down the sides as necessary.
2. Adjust consistency: If the mixture is too thick, add a little more water (1 tablespoon at a time) until you reach your desired sorbet consistency.
3. Serve immediately: Scoop the sorbet into bowls and serve immediately for a soft-serve texture.
4. Optional freezing: For a firmer sorbet, transfer the mixture to an airtight container and freeze for an additional 1-2 hours before serving

COCONUT YOGURT WITH MANGO AND CHIA SEEDS

COOK TIME: **5 MIN**   SERVICE: **2 PERSONS**

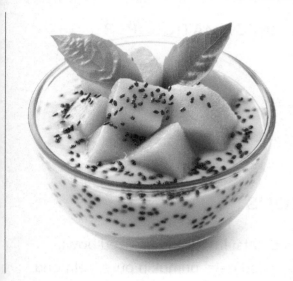

INGREDIENTS

- **1 cup unsweetened coconut yogurt**
- **1/2 cup fresh mango, diced**
- **2 tbsp chia seeds**
- **1 tsp honey or maple syrup (optional, for added sweetness)**
- **1 tbsp unsweetened shredded coconut (optional, for topping)**

NUTRITIONAL INFORMATION (PER SERVING)

- Protein: 4g
- Fat: 11g
- Carbohydrates: 17g
- Fiber: 6g
- Calories: 180 kcal

INSTRUCTIONS

1. Prepare the yogurt: In two serving bowls, divide the coconut yogurt evenly (1/2 cup per bowl).
2. Add the mango and chia seeds: Top each bowl with 1/4 cup diced mango and 1 tbsp chia seeds.
3. Optional sweetness: If you prefer extra sweetness, drizzle each bowl with 1/2 tsp honey or maple syrup.
4. Optional topping: For added texture, sprinkle 1/2 tbsp unsweetened shredded coconut over the top of each bowl.
5. Serve immediately: Enjoy this tropical, anti-inflammatory treat as a light snack or dessert.

PUMPKIN SPICE ENERGY BITES

COOK TIME: **10 MIN** (CHILL TIME 30 MIN)   SERVICE: **2 PERSONS**

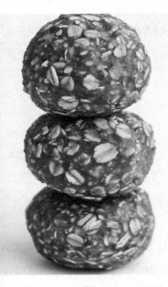

INGREDIENTS

- **1/2 cup rolled oats (gluten-free if needed)**
- **1/4 cup pumpkin purée (unsweetened)**
- **2 tbsp almond butter (or other nut butter)**
- **1 tbsp honey or maple syrup**
- **1/2 tsp pumpkin pie spice (or mix of cinnamon, nutmeg, ginger, and cloves)**
- **1/2 tsp vanilla extract**
- **1 tbsp chia seeds (optional, for extra fiber and omega-3s)**
- **Pinch of sea salt**

NUTRITIONAL INFORMATION (PER SERVING)

- Protein: 5g
- Fat: 8g
- Carbohydrates: 21g
- Fiber: 4g
- Calories: 160 kcal

INSTRUCTIONS

1. Mix the ingredients: In a medium-sized bowl, combine the rolled oats, pumpkin purée, almond butter, honey, pumpkin pie spice, vanilla extract, chia seeds (if using), and a pinch of sea salt. Stir until well combined and the mixture holds together.
2. Form into bites: Scoop about 1 tablespoon of the mixture at a time and roll it into small balls using your hands. You should get about 8-10 energy bites.
3. Chill: Place the energy bites on a plate and refrigerate for at least 30 minutes to firm up.
4. Serve: Enjoy the pumpkin spice energy bites as a quick, anti-inflammatory snack or dessert. Store any leftovers in an airtight container in the refrigerator for up to one week.

APPLE AND WALNUT CRUMBLE

COOK TIME: **30 MIN**   SERVICE: **2 PERSONS**

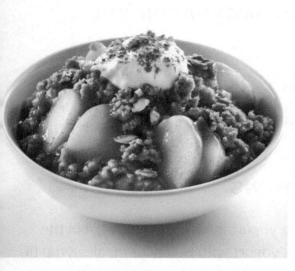

INGREDIENTS

For the Apple Filling:

- **2 medium apples (such as Granny Smith or Honeycrisp), peeled, cored, and sliced**
- **1 tbsp honey or maple syrup**
- **1/2 tsp cinnamon**
- **1/4 tsp ground ginger (optional, for extra anti-inflammatory benefits)**
- **1 tsp lemon juice**

For the Crumble Topping:

- **1/4 cup rolled oats (gluten-free if needed)**
- **1/4 cup chopped walnuts**
- **1 tbsp almond flour (or any other nut flour)**
- **1 tbsp coconut oil, melted**
- **1 tbsp honey or maple syrup**
- **Pinch of sea salt**

NUTRITIONAL INFORMATION (PER SERVING)

- Protein: 3g
- Fat: 12g
- Carbohydrates: 30g
- Fiber: 5g
- Calories: 220 kcal

INSTRUCTIONS

1. Preheat the oven: Preheat your oven to 350°F (175°C).
2. Prepare the apple filling: In a small bowl, toss the sliced apples with honey (or maple syrup), cinnamon, ground ginger, and lemon juice. Transfer the apple mixture into a small oven-safe dish.
3. Make the crumble topping: In a separate bowl, combine the oats, chopped walnuts, almond flour, melted coconut oil, honey (or maple syrup), and a pinch of sea salt. Mix until well combined and crumbly.
4. Assemble the crumble: Sprinkle the crumble topping evenly over the apple mixture in the dish.
5. Bake: Place the dish in the preheated oven and bake for 20-25 minutes, or until the apples are tender and the topping is golden brown.
6. Serve: Let the crumble cool slightly before serving. Enjoy it as a warm, anti-inflammatory dessert, or top it with a dollop of coconut yogurt for extra creaminess.

FROZEN YOGURT BARK WITH BLUEBERRIES AND ALMONDS

COOK TIME: 5 MIN (FREEZE TIME 180 MIN)   **SERVICE:** 2 PERSONS

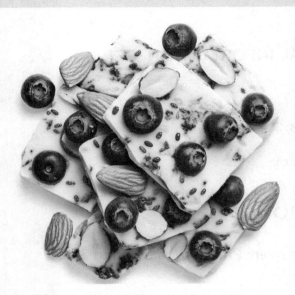

INGREDIENTS

- 1 cup plain Greek yogurt (unsweetened)
- 1 tbsp honey or maple syrup (optional, for sweetness)
- 1/4 cup fresh blueberries
- 2 tbsp sliced almonds
- 1 tsp chia seeds (optional, for added fiber and omega-3s)

NUTRITIONAL INFORMATION (PER SERVING)

- Protein: 8g
- Fat: 5g
- Carbohydrates: 17g
- Fiber: 3g
- Calories: 140 kcal

INSTRUCTIONS

1. Prepare the yogurt mixture: In a bowl, mix the plain Greek yogurt with honey or maple syrup (if using) until well combined.
2. Spread the yogurt: Line a baking sheet or tray with parchment paper. Spread the yogurt mixture evenly over the parchment paper, about 1/4-inch thick.
3. Add toppings: Sprinkle the blueberries, sliced almonds, and chia seeds (if using) evenly over the yogurt.
4. Freeze: Place the tray in the freezer for at least 2-3 hours, or until the yogurt is fully frozen and firm.
5. Break into pieces: Once frozen, remove the yogurt bark from the tray and break it into bite-sized pieces.
6. Serve: Enjoy immediately or store the frozen yogurt bark in an airtight container in the freezer for up to one week.

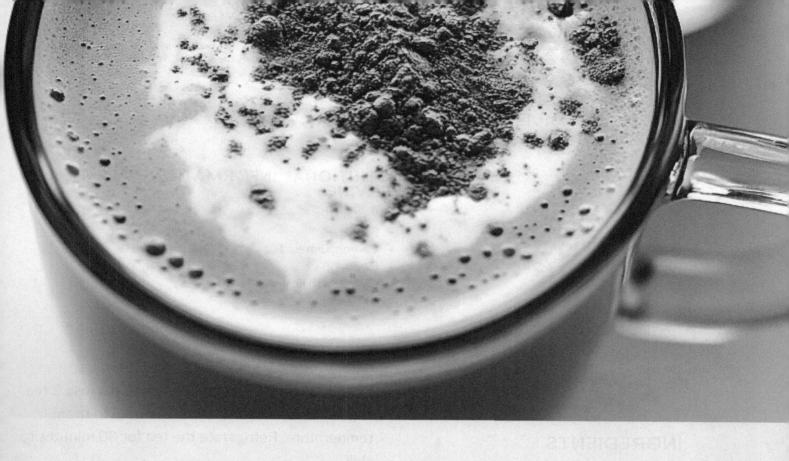

Beverages

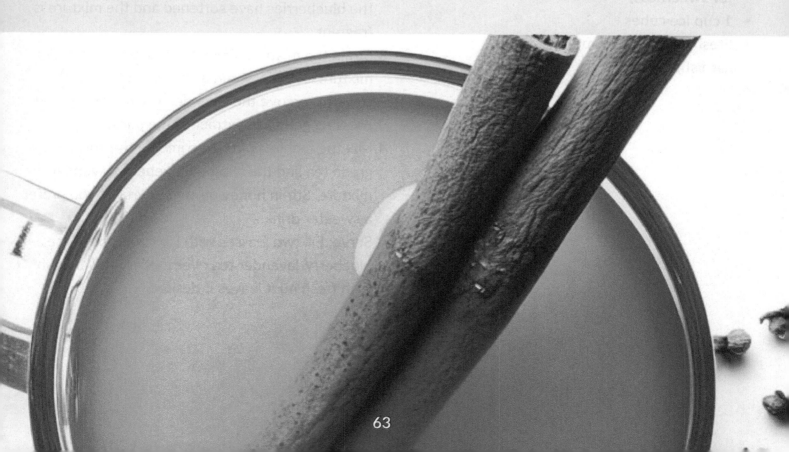

BLUEBERRY AND LAVENDER ICED TEA

COOK TIME: 5 MIN (CHILL TIME 30 MIN) SERVICE: 2 PERSONS

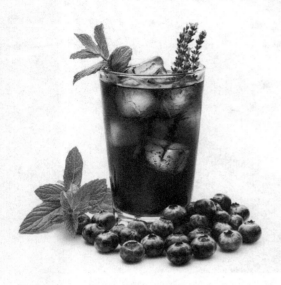

INGREDIENTS

- 1/2 cup fresh or frozen blueberries
- 2 tsp dried lavender
- 2 cups brewed green tea (chilled)
- 1 tsp honey or maple syrup (optional for sweetness)
- 1 cup ice cubes
- Fresh mint leaves (optional, for garnish)
-

NUTRITIONAL INFORMATION (PER SERVING)

- Protein: 0g
- Fat: 0g
- Carbohydrates: 10g
- Fiber: 1g
- Calories: 40 kcal

INSTRUCTIONS

1. Brew the tea: Brew 2 cups of green tea (use 2 tea bags or loose tea) and allow it to cool to room temperature. Refrigerate the tea for 30 minutes to chill.
2. Prepare the blueberry-lavender mixture: In a small saucepan, combine the blueberries, dried lavender, and 1/4 cup of water. Bring to a simmer over medium heat and cook for 5-7 minutes, until the blueberries have softened and the mixture is fragrant.
3. Strain the mixture: Once the blueberry-lavender mixture is ready, strain it through a fine-mesh sieve to remove the lavender and blueberry skins, pressing gently to extract all the juice.
4. Mix the tea: In a pitcher, combine the chilled green tea and the strained blueberry-lavender mixture. Stir in honey or maple syrup if you prefer a sweeter drink.
5. Serve: Fill two glasses with ice cubes, pour the blueberry-lavender tea over the ice, and garnish with fresh mint leaves if desired.

CINNAMON AND CLOVE SPICED CIDER

COOK TIME: **20 MIN**   SERVICE: **2 PERSONS**

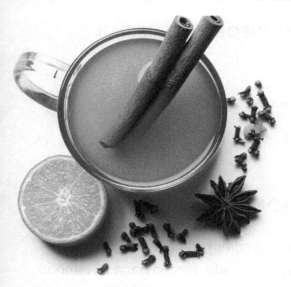

INGREDIENTS

- **2 cups apple cider (unsweetened)**
- **1 cinnamon stick**
- **4-5 whole cloves**
- **1/2 tsp ground ginger (optional for extra anti-inflammatory benefits)**
- **1 tsp honey or maple syrup (optional, for sweetness)**
- **1 orange slice (optional, for garnish)**

NUTRITIONAL INFORMATION (PER SERVING)

- Protein: 0g
- Fat: 0g
- Carbohydrates: 30g
- Fiber: 0g
- Calories: 120 kca

INSTRUCTIONS

1. Combine the ingredients: In a small saucepan, add the apple cider, cinnamon stick, whole cloves, and ground ginger (if using).
2. Simmer: Heat the mixture over medium heat until it starts to simmer. Lower the heat and allow it to simmer gently for 10-15 minutes to let the flavors meld.
3. Strain the cider: Remove the cinnamon stick and cloves by straining the cider through a fine-mesh sieve.
4. Add sweetness (optional): Stir in the honey or maple syrup if you'd like to sweeten the cider.
5. Serve: Pour the spiced cider into mugs and garnish with an orange slice, if desired. Serve warm.

SPINACH AND AVOCADO GREEN SMOOTHIE

COOK TIME: 5 MIN   SERVICE: 2 PERSONS

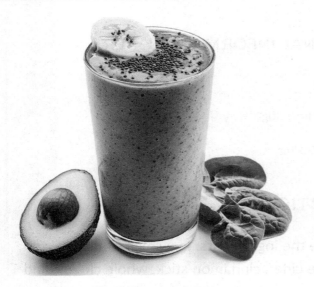

NUTRITIONAL INFORMATION (PER SERVING)

- Protein: 4g
- Fat: 10g
- Carbohydrates: 15g
- Fiber: 7g
- Calories: 170 kcal

INGREDIENTS

- **1 cup fresh spinach**
- **1/2 ripe avocado**
- **1/2 banana (frozen for extra creaminess)**
- **1 cup almond milk (unsweetened)**
- **1/2 cup water (or more for desired consistency)**
- **1 tbsp chia seeds (optional, for extra fiber and omega-3s)**
- **1 tsp honey or maple syrup (optional, for sweetness)**
- **1/2 tsp ground flaxseeds (optional, for extra anti-inflammatory benefits)**

INSTRUCTIONS

1. Prepare the ingredients: In a blender, add the fresh spinach, avocado, frozen banana, almond milk, water, chia seeds (if using), honey or maple syrup (if using), and ground flaxseeds (if using).
2. Blend: Blend on high speed until smooth and creamy. Add more water or almond milk if a thinner consistency is desired.
3. Serve: Divide the smoothie into two glasses and enjoy immediately as a nutrient-packed, anti-inflammatory breakfast or snack.

CRANBERRY AND ORANGE SPARKLING WATER

COOK TIME: **5 MIN**   SERVICE: **2 PERSONS**

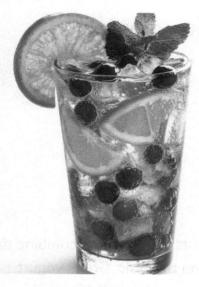

INGREDIENTS

- **1/2 cup unsweetened cranberry juice (pure cranberry juice)**
- **1/2 cup sparkling water**
- **Juice of 1 orange**
- **1-2 orange slices (for garnish)**
- **Fresh mint leaves (optional, for garnish)**
- **1 tsp honey or maple syrup (optional, for sweetness)**

NUTRITIONAL INFORMATION (PER SERVING)

- Protein: 0g
- Fat: 0g
- Carbohydrates: 12g
- Fiber: 0g
- Calories: 50 kcal

INSTRUCTIONS

1. Mix the juices: In a small pitcher, combine the unsweetened cranberry juice and the freshly squeezed orange juice. Stir in honey or maple syrup if you'd like extra sweetness.
2. Add sparkling water: Pour the cranberry-orange mixture into two glasses filled with ice, then top each glass with sparkling water.
3. Garnish and serve: Add a slice of orange and a few fresh mint leaves for garnish. Serve immediately and enjoy this refreshing anti-inflammatory beverage.

MANGO TURMERIC LASSI

COOK TIME: **5 MIN**   SERVICE: **2 PERSONS**

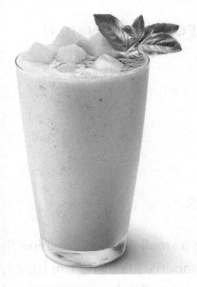

INGREDIENTS

- **1/2 cup fresh or frozen mango chunks**
- **1/2 tsp ground turmeric**
- **1/2 cup plain Greek yogurt (or dairy-free yogurt for vegan option)**
- **1/2 cup almond milk (unsweetened)**
- **1 tsp honey or maple syrup (optional, for sweetness)**
- **1/4 tsp ground ginger (optional, for extra anti-inflammatory benefits)**
- **1/2 tsp ground cinnamon (optional, for added flavor)**
- **Ice cubes (optional, for a chilled version)**

NUTRITIONAL INFORMATION (PER SERVING)

- Protein: 6g
- Fat: 4g
- Carbohydrates: 18g
- Fiber: 2g
- Calories: 120 kcal

INSTRUCTIONS

1. Prepare the ingredients: In a blender, combine the mango chunks, ground turmeric, Greek yogurt, almond milk, honey or maple syrup (if using), ground ginger, and ground cinnamon (if using).
2. Blend: Blend on high speed until smooth and creamy. If desired, add a few ice cubes for a chilled version and blend again until smooth.
3. Serve: Divide the mango turmeric lassi into two glasses and enjoy immediately.

MATCHA GREEN TEA LATTE

COOK TIME: **5 MIN**   SERVICE: **2 PERSONS**

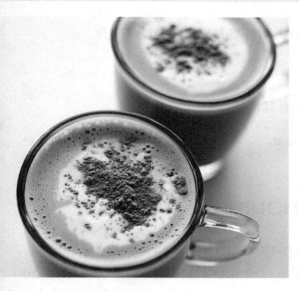

INGREDIENTS

- **2 tsp matcha green tea powder**
- **1 cup almond milk (unsweetened, or any plant-based milk)**
- **1 cup water (hot but not boiling)**
- **1 tsp honey or maple syrup (optional, for sweetness)**
- **1/2 tsp vanilla extract (optional, for added flavor)**

NUTRITIONAL INFORMATION (PER SERVING)

- Protein: 2g
- Fat: 3g
- Carbohydrates: 5g
- Fiber: 1g
- Calories: 50 kcal

INSTRUCTIONS

1. Prepare the matcha: In a small bowl, whisk the matcha green tea powder with 1/2 cup hot water until smooth and no lumps remain. Use a bamboo whisk or electric frother for best results.
2. Heat the milk: In a small saucepan, heat the almond milk over medium heat until warm, but not boiling. If using vanilla extract, stir it into the milk as it heats.
3. Combine the tea and milk: Divide the whisked matcha between two mugs. Add the remaining hot water and the warmed almond milk to each mug, stirring gently to combine.
4. Sweeten: Add honey or maple syrup if desired, and stir well.
5. Serve: Enjoy immediately as a warm, calming, anti-inflammatory beverage.

CHIA SEED LEMONADE

COOK TIME: 5 MIN (SOAK TIME 15 MIN)   **SERVICE:** 2 PERSONS

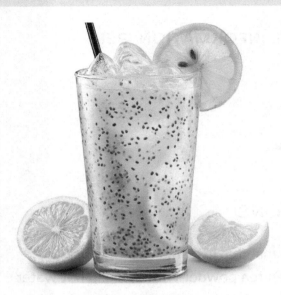

NUTRITIONAL INFORMATION (PER SERVING)

- Protein: 2g
- Fat: 2g
- Carbohydrates: 10g
- Fiber: 5g
- Calories: 60 kcal

INGREDIENTS

- **1 tbsp chia seeds**
- **2 cups water**
- **2 tbsp fresh lemon juice (from about 1 lemon)**
- **1 tbsp honey or maple syrup (optional, for sweetness)**
- **Ice cubes (optional, for serving)**
- **Lemon slices (optional, for garnish)**

INSTRUCTIONS

1. Soak the chia seeds: In a small bowl or jar, combine the chia seeds and 1/4 cup of water. Stir well and let the chia seeds soak for about 10-15 minutes until they form a gel-like consistency.
2. Prepare the lemonade: In a separate pitcher, mix the remaining water, fresh lemon juice, and honey or maple syrup (if using). Stir until the honey is dissolved.
3. Combine: Once the chia seeds have soaked, add them to the lemonade mixture and stir well to combine.
4. Serve: Divide the chia lemonade between two glasses, adding ice cubes if desired. Garnish with lemon slices for a fresh touch.

BEETROOT AND CARROT JUICE

COOK TIME: **5 MIN**   SERVICE: **2 PERSONS**

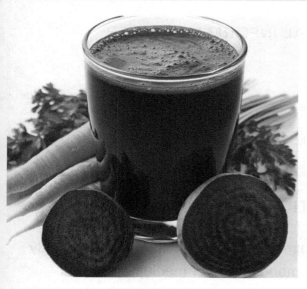

INGREDIENTS

- **1 medium beet (peeled and chopped)**
- **2 medium carrots (peeled and chopped)**
- **1/2 apple (optional, for sweetness)**
- **1-inch piece of fresh ginger (optional, for extra anti-inflammatory benefits)**
- **1 cup water (or more, as needed)**

NUTRITIONAL INFORMATION (PER SERVING)

- Protein: 1g
- Fat: 0g
- Carbohydrates: 20g
- Fiber: 3g (if unstrained)
- Calories: 80 kcal

INSTRUCTIONS

1. Prepare the ingredients: Peel and chop the beet, carrots, and apple (if using) into small pieces that can fit into your blender or juicer.
2. Juicing method:
3. In a juicer: Run the beet, carrots, apple, and ginger through your juicer. Add water if needed to adjust the consistency.
4. In a blender: If using a blender, add the beet, carrots, apple, ginger, and water. Blend until smooth. Strain the mixture through a fine mesh sieve or cheesecloth to remove the pulp, if desired.
5. Serve: Pour the juice into two glasses and enjoy immediately for the best flavor and nutritional benefits.

CINNAMON-SPICED ALMOND MILK

COOK TIME: **10 MIN**   SERVICE: **2 PERSONS**

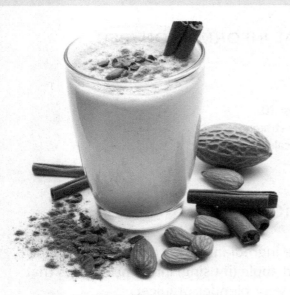

NUTRITIONAL INFORMATION (PER SERVING)

- Protein: 1g
- Fat: 3g
- Carbohydrates: 5g
- Fiber: 1g
- Calories: 40 kcal

INGREDIENTS

- **2 cups almond milk (unsweetened)**
- **1/2 tsp ground cinnamon**
- **1/4 tsp ground ginger (optional, for extra anti-inflammatory benefits)**
- **1 tsp honey or maple syrup (optional, for sweetness)**
- **1/2 tsp vanilla extract (optional, for added flavor)**
- **Pinch of sea salt (optional)**

INSTRUCTIONS

1. Heat the almond milk: In a small saucepan, gently heat the almond milk over medium heat until warm but not boiling.
2. Add spices and sweeteners: Stir in the ground cinnamon, ginger (if using), honey or maple syrup (if using), vanilla extract, and a pinch of sea salt. Whisk until well combined and the spices are evenly distributed.
3. Simmer: Reduce the heat to low and simmer for 3-5 minutes, allowing the flavors to meld.
4. Serve: Pour the spiced almond milk into two mugs and enjoy immediately as a warm, comforting anti-inflammatory beverage.

TART CHERRY JUICE

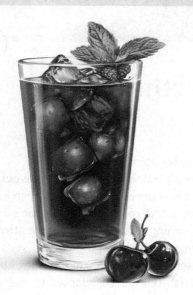

NUTRITIONAL INFORMATION (PER SERVING)

- Protein: 0g
- Fat: 0g
- Carbohydrates: 15g
- Fiber: 0g
- Calories: 60 kcal

INSTRUCTIONS

1. Mix the ingredients: In a small pitcher, combine the tart cherry juice and water. Stir in honey or maple syrup if you prefer a sweeter taste.
2. Serve: Divide the tart cherry juice mixture between two glasses filled with ice cubes.
3. Garnish: Optionally, garnish with fresh mint leaves for a refreshing touch.

INGREDIENTS

- **1/2 cup unsweetened tart cherry juice (pure concentrate)**
- **1/2 cup water**
- **1 tsp honey or maple syrup (optional, for sweetness)**
- **Ice cubes (optional, for serving)**
- **Fresh mint leaves (optional, for garnish)**

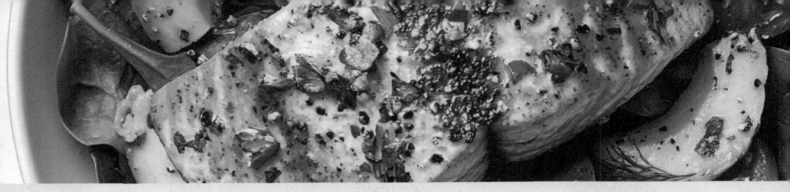

Lifestyle Tips for Managing Arthritis

Managing arthritis requires a holistic approach that goes beyond medication and diet. Integrating healthy lifestyle habits, like regular exercise, stress management, and mindful eating, can significantly improve the quality of life for those with arthritis. This chapter explores these key aspects of an arthritis-friendly lifestyle, tailored for people in the USA.

1. Incorporating Exercise and Movement

Regular physical activity is vital for managing arthritis, as it helps maintain joint mobility, build muscle strength, and reduce stiffness. In the USA, with access to parks, fitness centers, and community activities, integrating movement into daily life is achievable with the right approach.

A. Low-Impact Exercises for Joint Health

For people with arthritis, high-impact exercises may cause discomfort. Instead, low-impact exercises provide a way to stay active without overburdening the joints:

- Walking: A brisk walk in the neighborhood or a local park can help improve circulation, maintain joint flexibility, and boost mood.
- Swimming or Aquatic Exercise: Water-based activities are especially helpful for arthritis sufferers because the water supports your weight, reducing stress on joints while allowing for full-body movement.
- Cycling: Whether on a stationary bike or a road bike, cycling strengthens muscles around the knees and hips, supporting joint health.

Yoga and Tai Chi: These gentle practices improve flexibility, balance, and overall joint health. Many community centers and online platforms in the USA offer arthritis-friendly yoga and Tai Chi classes.

B. Strength Training for Joint Support

Incorporating strength training, 2-3 times per week, can strengthen muscles and provide more support to joints:

- Resistance Bands: Use resistance bands for gentle muscle strengthening exercises. Bands are affordable and easy to use at home or on the go.
- Bodyweight Exercises: Exercises like squats, lunges, and modified push-ups can be adapted to suit various fitness levels and help build muscle strength around joints.
- Light Weight Lifting: Start with lighter weights to avoid straining your joints, focusing on exercises that strengthen core muscles, legs, and arms.

C. Daily Movement and Stretching

Incorporating simple stretches into your daily routine can increase flexibility and reduce stiffness:

- Morning Stretching Routine: Start the day with a gentle stretch, focusing on the hips, back, shoulders, and legs to loosen up joints after sleep.
- Active Breaks: Set reminders to stand, stretch, and walk throughout the day, especially if you have a desk job. Incorporating movement helps reduce joint stiffness.

"Eat to heal—every bite brings you closer to a stronger, healthier you."

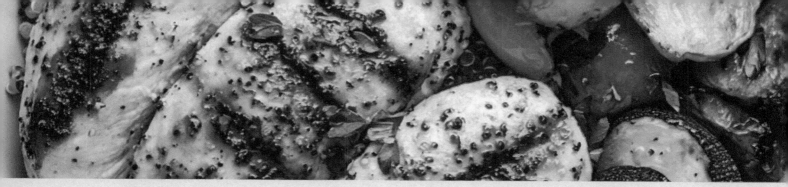

Stress Management Techniques

Stress can worsen the symptoms of arthritis by increasing inflammation in the body. Effectively managing stress is key to reducing flare-ups and maintaining a balanced, healthy lifestyle.

A. Mindfulness and Meditation

Mindfulness practices, such as meditation, have been shown to reduce stress and inflammation:

- Guided Meditation: Many apps in the USA, like Calm and Headspace, offer guided meditations designed to relieve stress. A 10-minute session in the morning or before bed can help manage anxiety.
- Deep Breathing Exercises: Simple deep breathing techniques can be done anywhere to help manage stress. Try the 4-7-8 breathing technique—inhale for 4 seconds, hold for 7 seconds, and exhale for 8 seconds.
- Body Scan Meditation: Lie down in a comfortable position and focus on each part of your body, bringing awareness and relaxation to every muscle group. This can help relieve tension in joints.

B. Relaxation Techniques

Incorporating relaxation into your routine can alleviate stress:

- Massage Therapy: Many clinics in the USA offer specialized massages for people with arthritis to reduce muscle tension around the joints.
- Aromatherapy: Use calming essential oils like lavender, chamomile, or eucalyptus in a diffuser or added to a warm bath to promote relaxation.
- Hot and Cold Therapy: Applying heat to stiff joints (like with heating pads or warm baths) and cold packs to inflamed areas can provide relief and promote relaxation.

C. Connecting with Support Networks

Having a community is essential for stress relief:

- Support Groups: Joining arthritis support groups, either in-person or online, provides emotional support and practical advice. Organizations like the Arthritis Foundation offer valuable resources.
- Therapy and Counseling: Speaking to a therapist can help manage the emotional aspects of arthritis. Many telehealth services in the USA make accessing counseling easier than ever.

"Fuel your body with goodness, and it will thank you every day."

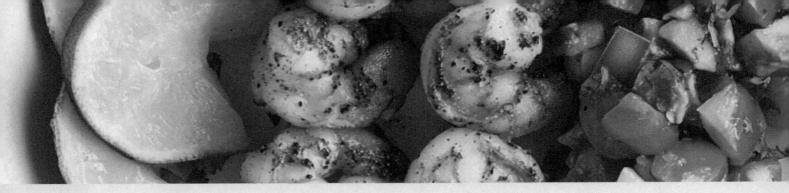

Mindful Eating Practices

Eating mindfully can help reduce inflammation, promote digestion, and enhance the overall experience of eating for those managing arthritis.

A. Savoring Anti-Inflammatory Foods

Mindful eating begins with selecting anti-inflammatory foods and savoring each bite:

- **Whole Foods**: Focus on consuming whole foods like fruits, vegetables, lean proteins, and whole grains, all of which support joint health and reduce inflammation.
- **Eat Slowly**: Take time to chew thoroughly and appreciate the flavors of your meal. This practice promotes better digestion and allows you to tune in to hunger and fullness cues.
- **Portion Control**: Mindful portion control can help maintain a healthy weight, reducing stress on the **joints. Consider using smaller plates or paying attention to portion sizes.**

B. Meal Planning for Arthritis

Planning your meals ahead of time can ensure you're getting the nutrients you need while reducing the stress of daily decision-making:

- **Prep Anti-Inflammatory Meals**: Batch-cook meals high in antioxidants, omega-3s, and fiber. For example, prepare a large pot of vegetable soup or roasted salmon for the week.
- **Snack Mindfully**: Choose snacks rich in healthy fats, such as nuts, seeds, and avocado. Pack portable snacks when on the go to avoid processed foods.

C. Hydration

Staying hydrated is crucial for joint lubrication and overall health:

- **Drink Water Throughout the Day**: Aim to drink 8 cups of water a day. Carry a reusable water bottle with you as a reminder.
- **Infused Water**: Add slices of lemon, cucumber, or berries to your water for extra flavor and antioxidants.

"Eat better, feel better, live better."

Made in the USA
Las Vegas, NV
30 December 2024

15595032R00044